Knee-deep in Pandemia:
Plague Doctor Illustrations for the 21st Century

Kurt Mitchell

ed. Daividh Eideard Mitchell

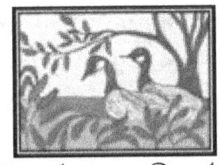

Riverhaven Books

Knee-deep in Pandemia: Plague Doctor Illustrations for the 21st Century is a work of art. Some creative license was taken by the artist in his creation of these works.

Published in the United States by Riverhaven Books, Massachusetts.

ISBN: 978-1-951854-15-7

Printed in the United States of America

Edited by Daividh Eideard Mitchell
Designed by Stephanie Lynn Blackman
Whitman, MA

To the doctors and nurses who have served on the front lines during the awful COVID-19 pandemic

Table of Contents

Foreword

~ Wendy Miller

Plague Doctor?
What?
Kurt, how did you come up with that?

Kurt Mitchell (1952-2020) was an artist who never left home without his sketchbook and black pens in his pocket. He could often be found at Horse Thief Hollow microbrewery in the Beverly Hills-Morgan Park area of Chicago, drawing at his table in "Kurt's corner," or at the bar. He made many friends and drew many sketches there on anything he could get a hold of, from his sketchbooks to cocktail napkins.Kurt and I had been friends since the age of two. In all that time, his wit and creativity never ceased to amaze me. We were in and out of touch at times, but always remained in contact--always able to pick up without missing a beat--like really close cousins.

We both lived in Cook County, Illinois which, due to the spread of the COVID-19 virus, SHUT DOWN on March 16, 2020. Restaurants and bars were closed until Phase 4. So, from March 16 until

June 24, Kurt's lifelines to the world were his phone and his pen.

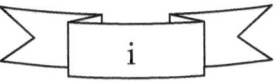

Kurt and I talked on the phone a lot during this time. I often called him while I was walking my Golden Retriever in our neighborhood so he could come down for a "social distanced" visit and a "dog fix." I specifically remember talking to him the day that he drew "Close the Damn Door." It was the only time he didn't come down to chat because he was so intent on uploading that sketch to colorize for a projected poster before he finished the pen-and-ink portion. Art trumped a Golden Retriever!

During our many conversations we often talked about what was happening in the world and his ideas for the Plague Doctor drawings:

• People were hoarding toilet paper- so was the Plague Doctor ("Plague Joker").

• People were drinking a lot- Plague Doctor had trouble with that ("Drinking Problem")!

• People were arguing over wearing a mask- Plague Doctor had that covered (and uncovered).

• People were protesting peacefully and otherwise- Plague Doctor was involved in that too ("Something worth Burning" and "Heroic").

Famous works of art and literature were also referenced in the Plague Doctor as well as motion pictures. *Moby Dick* ("Call Me Ahab"), *The Exorcist* ("Out of the Fog") and even Miles Davis received a nod ("Pandemic Blues").

After Kurt's death his brother Jon and I went to his apartment to take care of some of those awful resultant details. I knew of the sketchbooks and had hoped against hope that we would find the one Kurt labelled "Book 04," which contained the Plague Doctor sketches. We found it, and it felt to me like finding the Holy Grail. Kurt held up a mirror to what we were all going through in this pandemic in this black-and-white pen-and-ink sketchbook.

"Plague Doctor? What? Kurt, how did you come up with that?"

I don't have an answer, but we are all the richer because he did.

Introduction

~ Daividh Eideard Mitchell

Kurt Davis Mitchell was my uncle. During his long and varied career as a freelance artist, illustrator, and writer, he worked on such diverse projects as *Jonah* and *Esther* from Chariot Books, Narnia-inspired board games for David C. Cook, his own beloved children's book *Poor Ralph*, and editorial cartoons for *The Chicago Reader*, *Chicago Tribune*, *Chicago Sun-Times*, *The Quill*, and others. For about twelve years, he also worked in video game development, contributing to such titles as *MechAssault* and *Septerra Core*. Then there was his later period of creativity, which largely consisted of self-published comics, graphic novels, greeting cards, and short stories. From here we have his comics *Cannonboy*, *Oxbluud*, and *The Pigeon Eater*, his anthropomorphic parable *Penguin's Progress*, his tongue-in-cheek *The Tao of Stubbie Pencil*, and his novel *A Stranger Side of Red*.

Growing up, I generally only saw my uncle during the holidays, but his work was a lasting presence in our household. Before I had seen any of his surreal pieces or editorial illustrations, we had our copies of *Poor Ralph*, *Esther,* and *Jonah*. The images in those works were burned into my head from an early age, of small characters dwarfed by their surroundings, and the brilliant little details that made these places seem hostile and intimidating even without their inhabitants, like the people in the wall painting who leer at Ralph as he passes by, or the stone cat faces carved into the archways of Cat Nineveh, looking down at Mouse Jonah as he tries to proclaim the message God has given him.

Yet it was Kurt's custom art that I remembered the most. Sometimes I even commissioned it myself. Waving my Imperial black and brown rubber Triceratops in the air, I suggested a concept that made sense only to five-year-old me: A Triceratops taking a bath! I watched in astonishment as he completed the illustration from where he sat at the kitchen table, using my Triceratops as a reference. The piece even included a cheesy joke: "Why did the Triceratops take a bath? Because he wanted to become ex-stinkt!"

And there were the custom T-shirts he supplied, of a tap-dancing Tyrannosaurus and a Mastodon wearing a striped shirt and eating a hot dog. Of course, the Christmas presents he brought over also tended to be cool things, like Dino-Riders and Teenage Mutant Ninja Turtles, which provided a much needed balance to the usual assortment of clothes and underwear.

Knowing Kurt as an adult proved even more rewarding as I explored my creative interests in college. As a budding writer I was always eager to share my fiction with him as he was sending us copies of *Cannonboy* and *Oxbluud*. Sadly, we never collaborated on anything, though the idea was brought up on at least one occasion.

I remember one night in which Kurt and I had a long and heartfelt conversation, discussing faith, politics, art, and pets. I listened as he told me with heartrending sincerity about the loss of his cat, about how

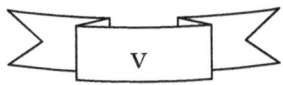

v

he had begun to pray with his cat when that impending loss became apparent, and how the cat had learned his routine of prayers and Psalm readings and began situating himself accordingly, as if he was reminding Kurt to pray.

"Dogs are your buddies, your pals," he told me. "Dogs touch your heart. But cats touch your soul. There's something spiritual about cats. The ancient Egyptians understood that."

It was such a fascinating observation that I felt compelled to use this line in a short story I wrote later on. A year or two later, when Kurt read the story, he said to me, "Wow, that was a great line. 'Dogs touch your heart, cats touch your soul.' Where did you get that from?"

I told him, of course, that he had said those exact words to me. He was astonished.

During his final years, Kurt remained productive despite the financial and professional setbacks he faced. His artistic output was a daily process, a honing of skills and a practiced labor of love that any artist should aspire toward. His *Morning Sky* series was a simple, daily rendering of the clouds above the treetops as he could see from his apartment, always the exact same vista, yet always interesting and unique.

What we have collected here is Kurt's very last artistic achievement: his own personal response to the COVID-19 pandemic through a series of surrealistic pen-and-ink illustrations. We have arranged them by date. Even when working within the confines of the Coronavirus lockdown in Chicago, Kurt found a creative way to

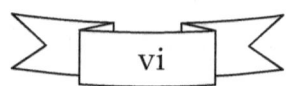

respond to the pandemic with wit, playfulness, pointed satire, and mordant humor. The setting, of course, is the world of 2020, but the fashion of choice is the mask of the 17th century physician.

In a pandemic, a mask is the only face you can present to the world. These plague doctors have *become* their work, so they are incorporeal beyond the strange light that shines through the eyeholes of their empty beaked masks. Sometimes they are figures of ambiguity, but far more often they are heroic, waging uphill battles against the dragon of COVID-19, floating puffer fishes their steeds or watch dogs, harpoons fashioned from their canes, and their hypodermics the lance of St. George.

Heroic doctors are, of course, what the world needs in the wake of a global pandemic. Kurt understood this fundamental truth, and expressed it with his trademark wit and style. It is our hope that you enjoy this collection of plague doctors both whimsical and beleaguered, and perhaps let them inspire you.

Prologue

During the Black Plague, certain people took care of the dying and the removal of the deceased. They were called "Plague Doctors" and they can be found in many historic works of art.

The elongated noses of the masks they wore contained mixtures of garlic and sweet essences in a vain attempt to ward off the disease and stench, and to ensure their anonymity.

~ Kurt Mitchell
March 16, 2020

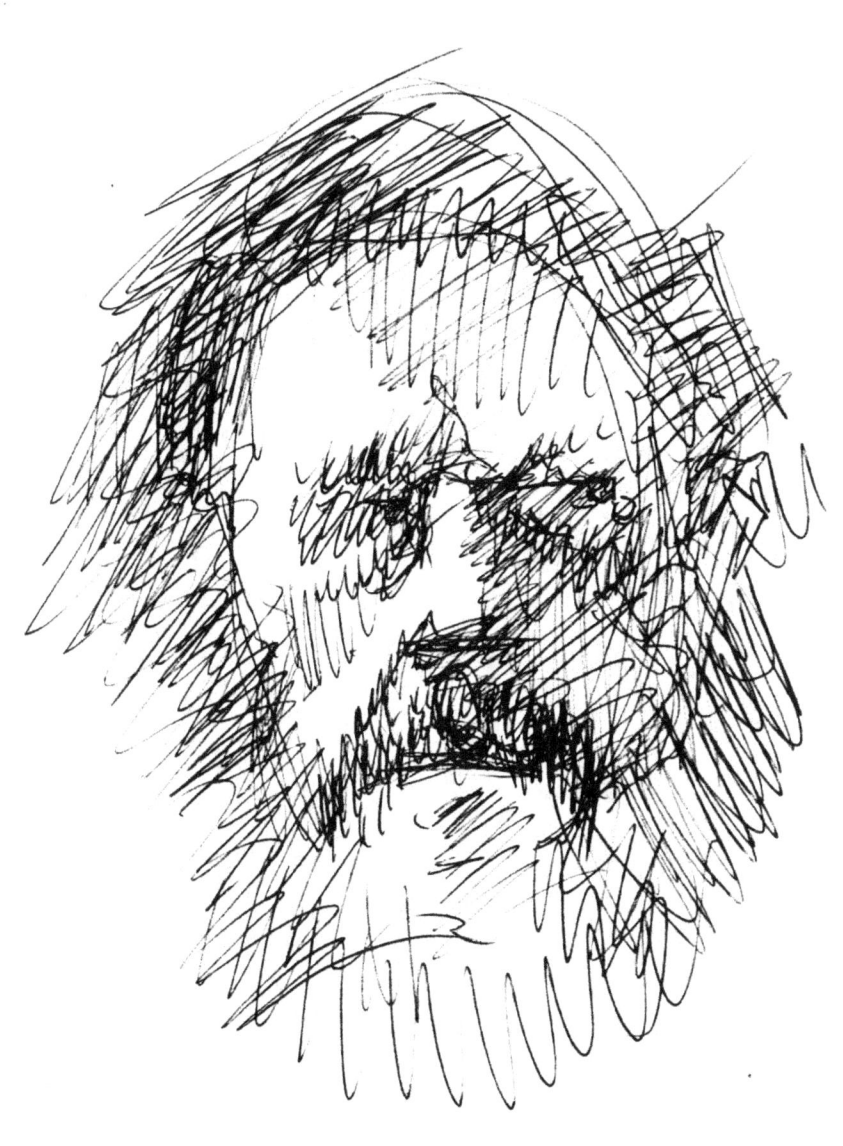

Kurt Mitchell: Self Portrait
March 19, 2019

The

Illustrations

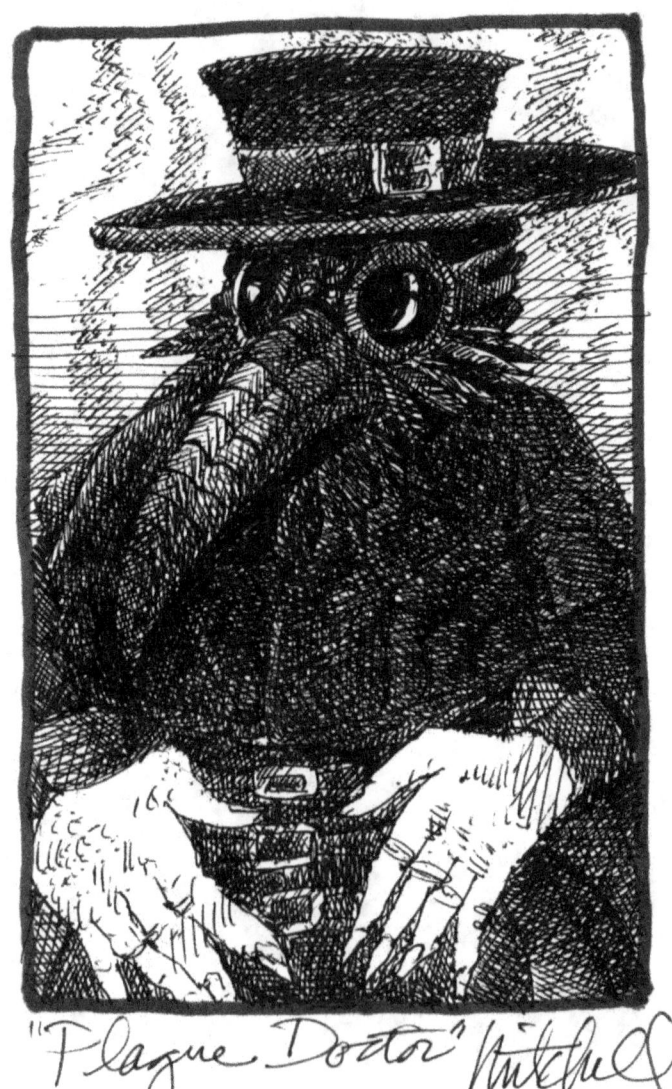

"Plague Doctor" Mitchell

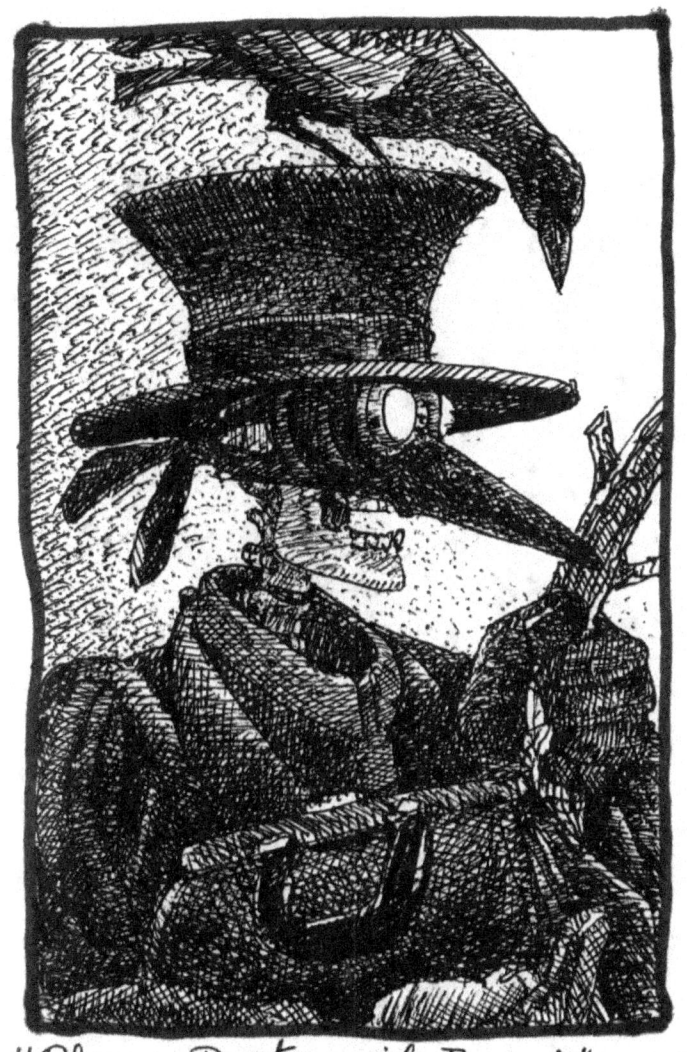

"Plague Doctor with Branch"

Mitchell

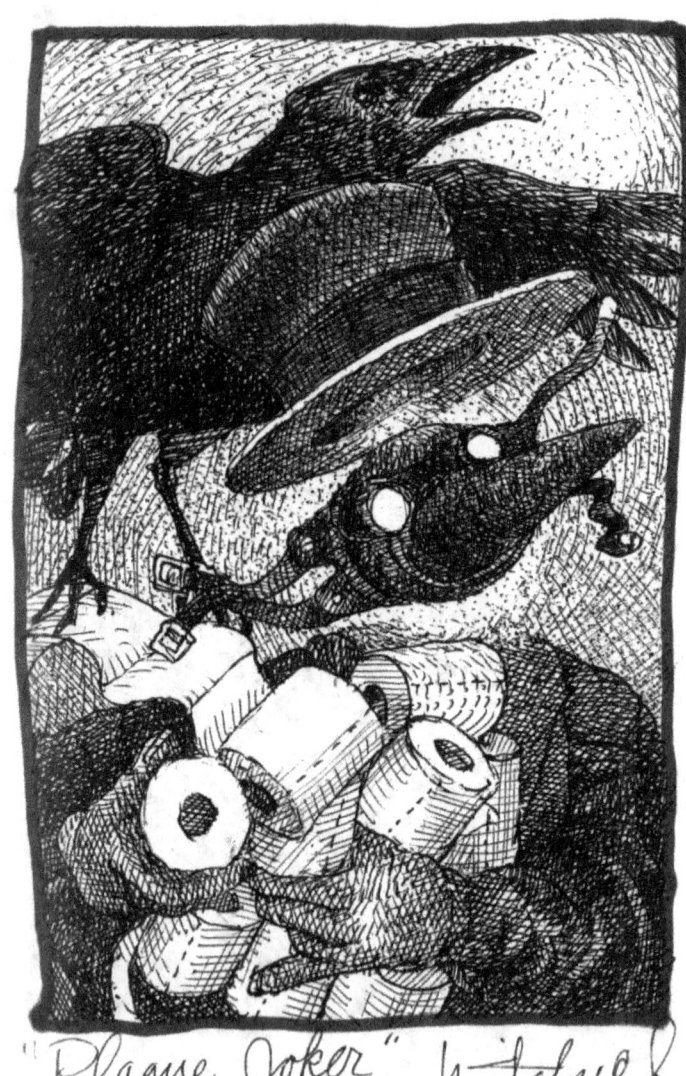

"Plague Joker" Mitchell

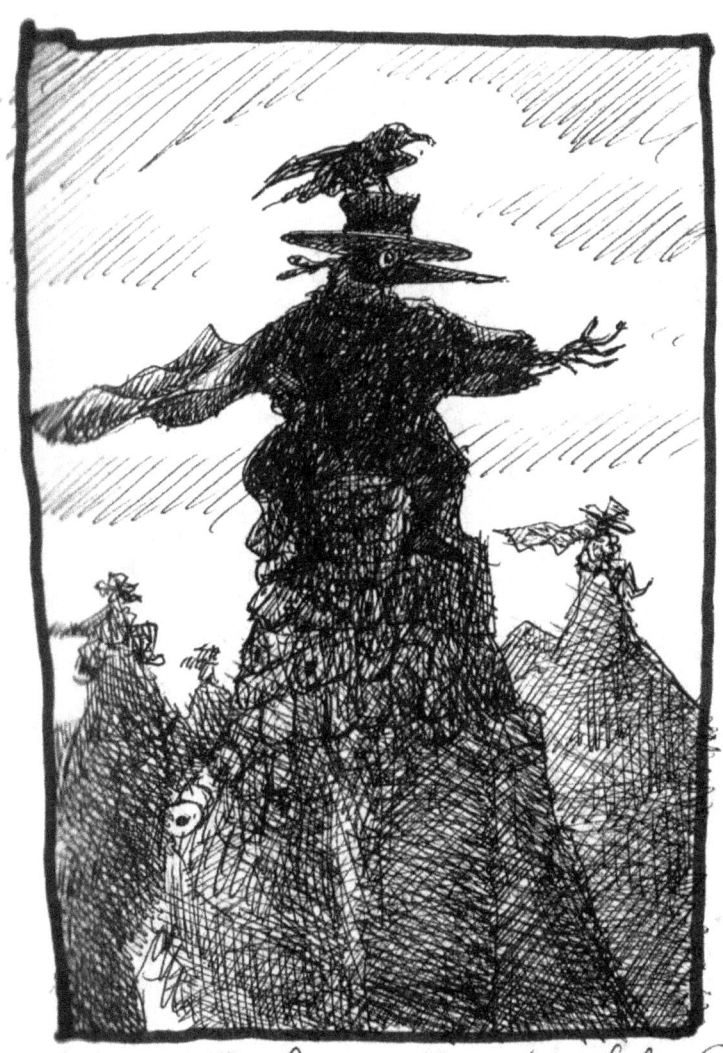

"Voluntary Quarantine"

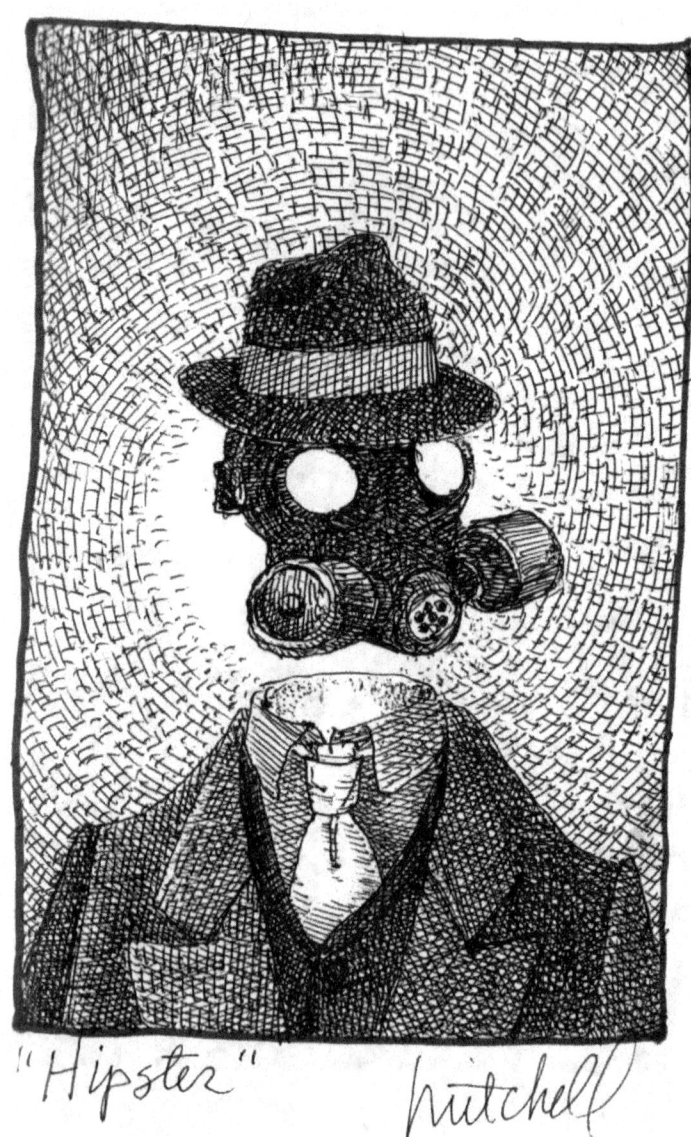

"Hipster"

mitchell

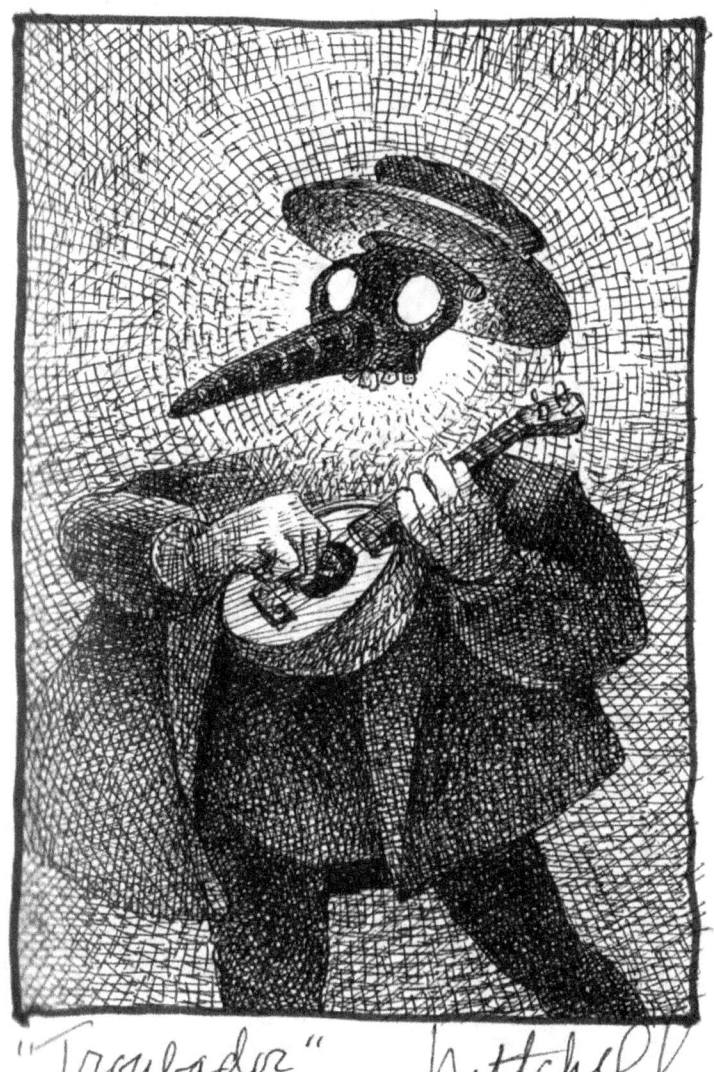

"Troubador"   Mitchell

March 18

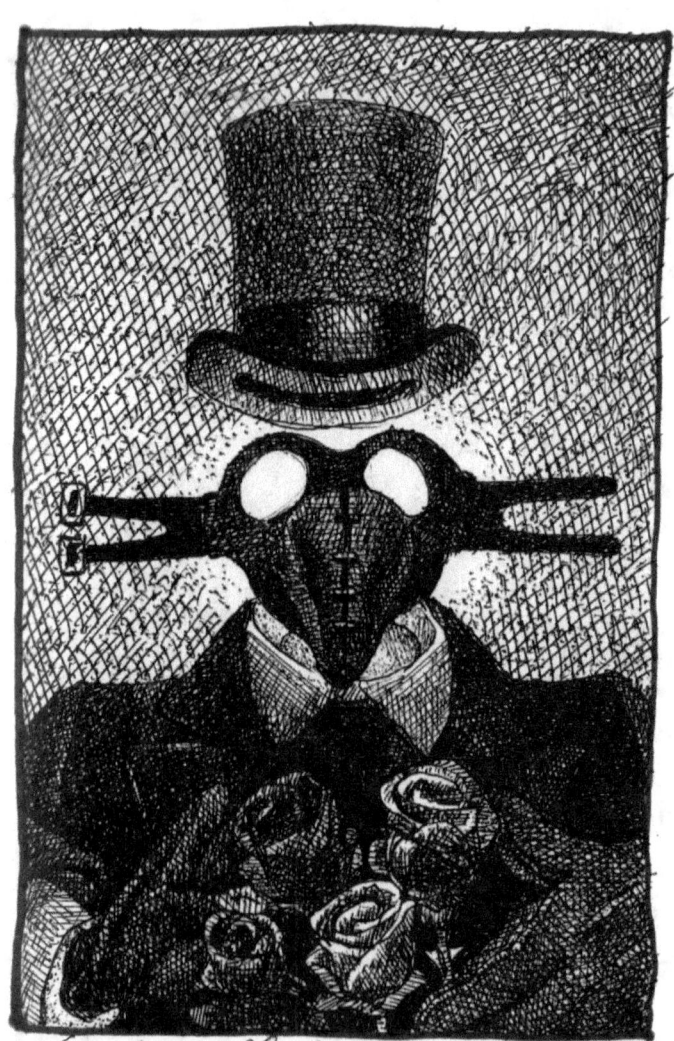

"Try To Smell The Roses"

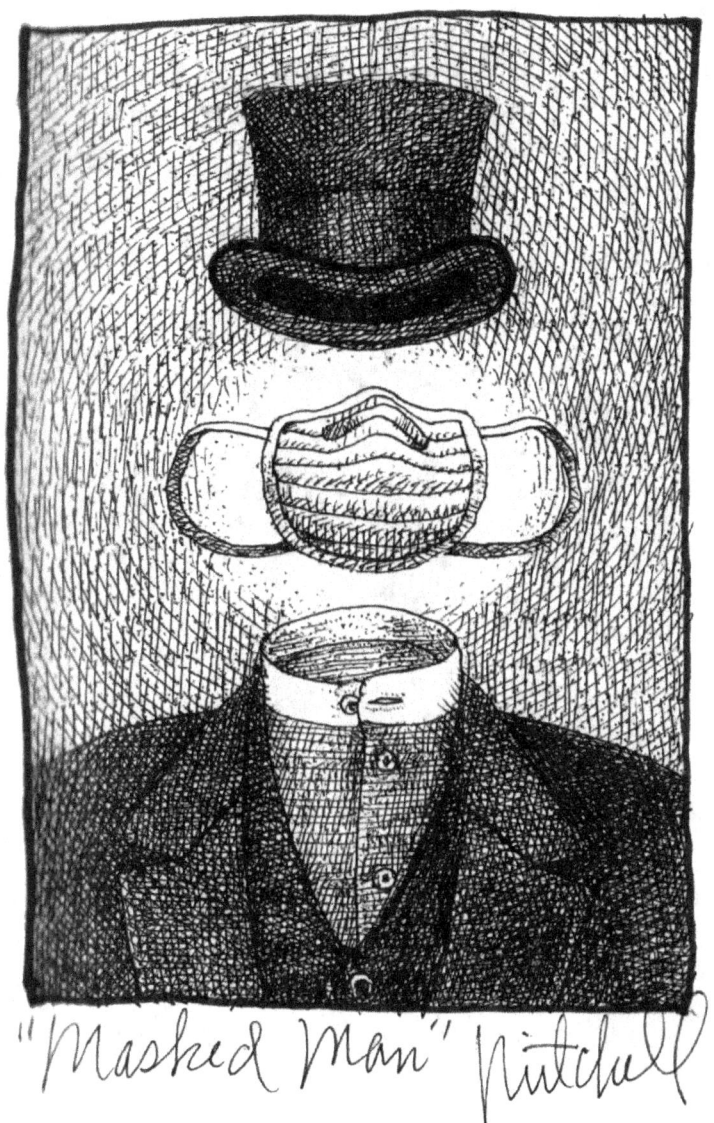

"Masked Man" Mitchell

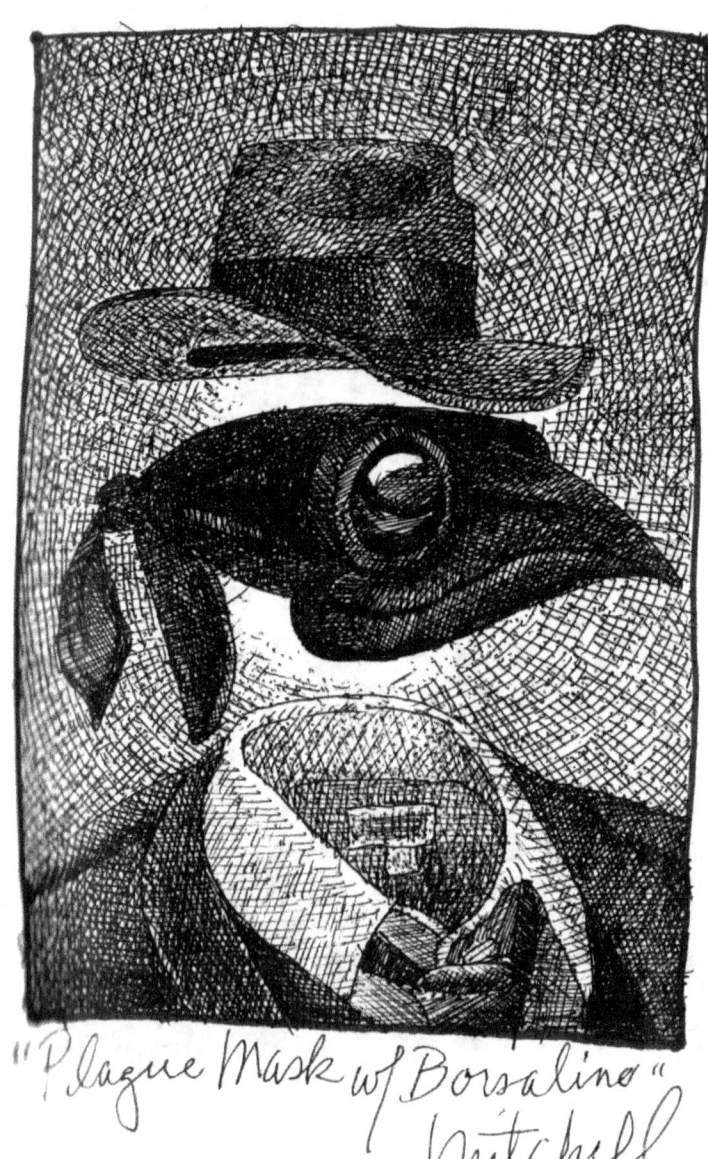

"Plague Mask w/ Borsalino"

Mitchell

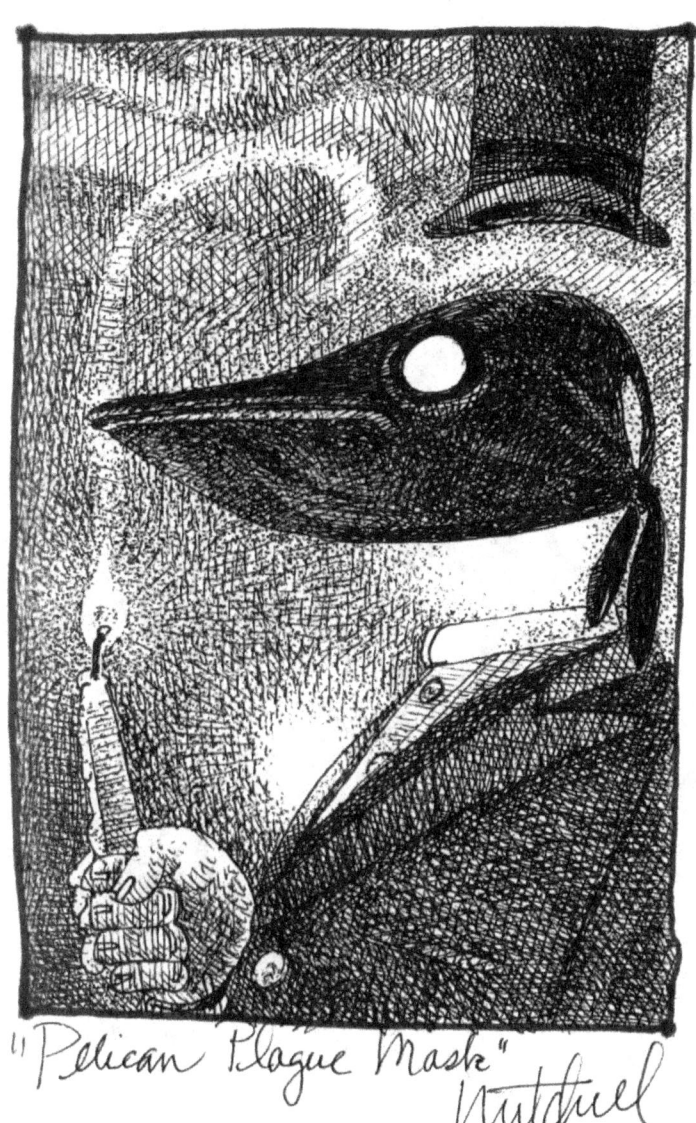

"Pelican "Plague Mask"

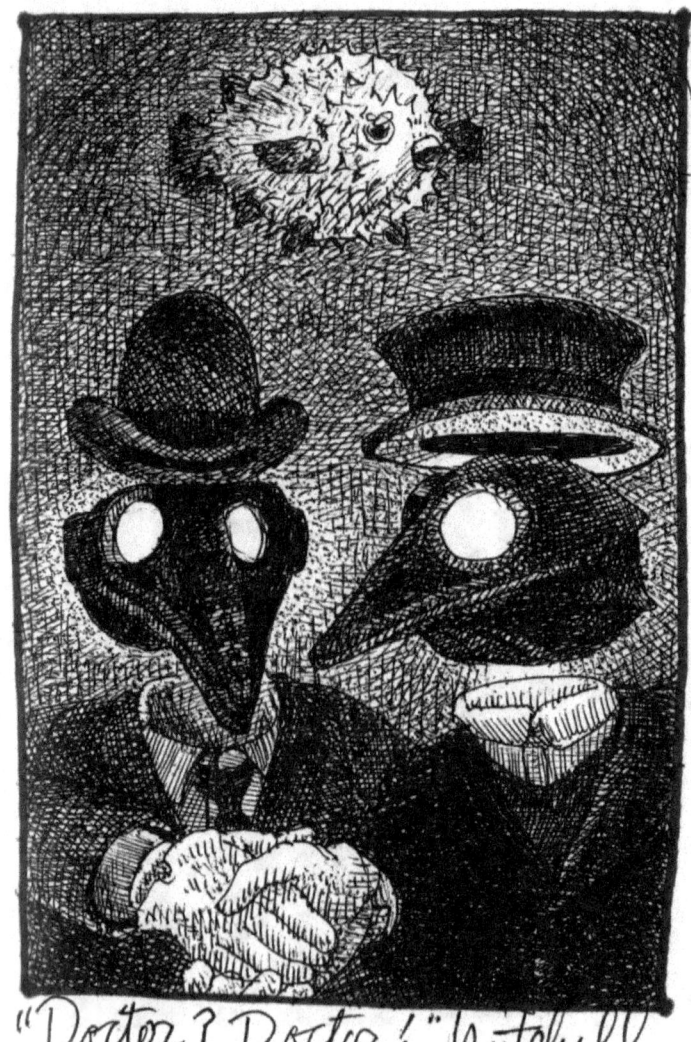

"Doctor? Doctor!" Pufferfish... Mitchell

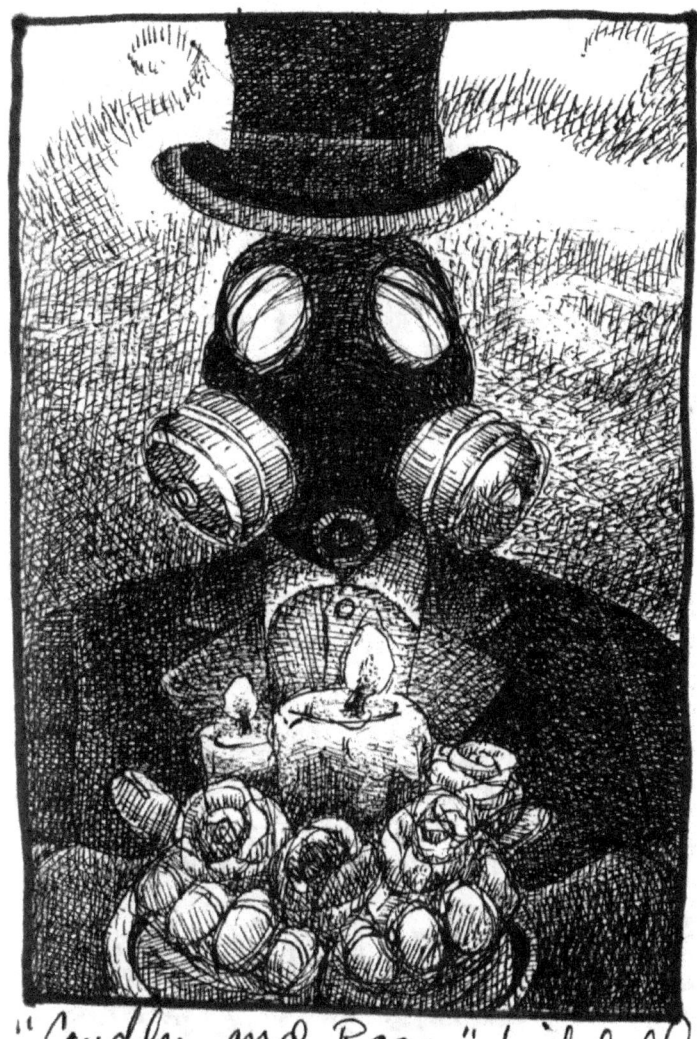

"Candles and Roses" Mitchell

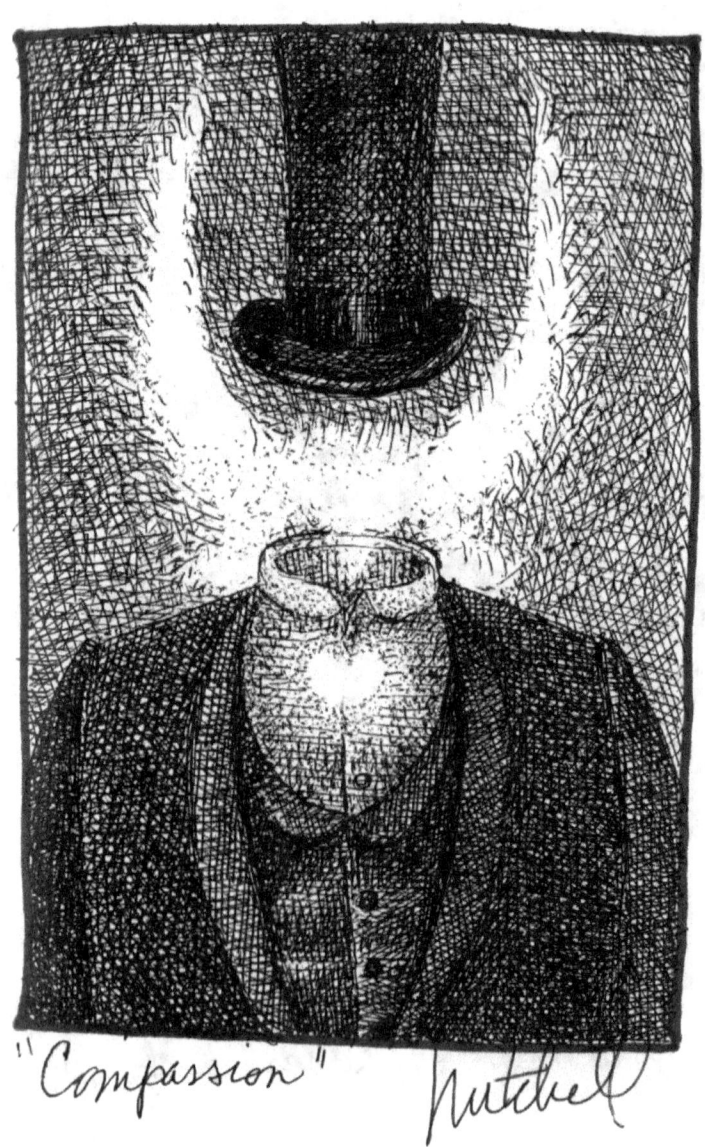

"*Compassion*"

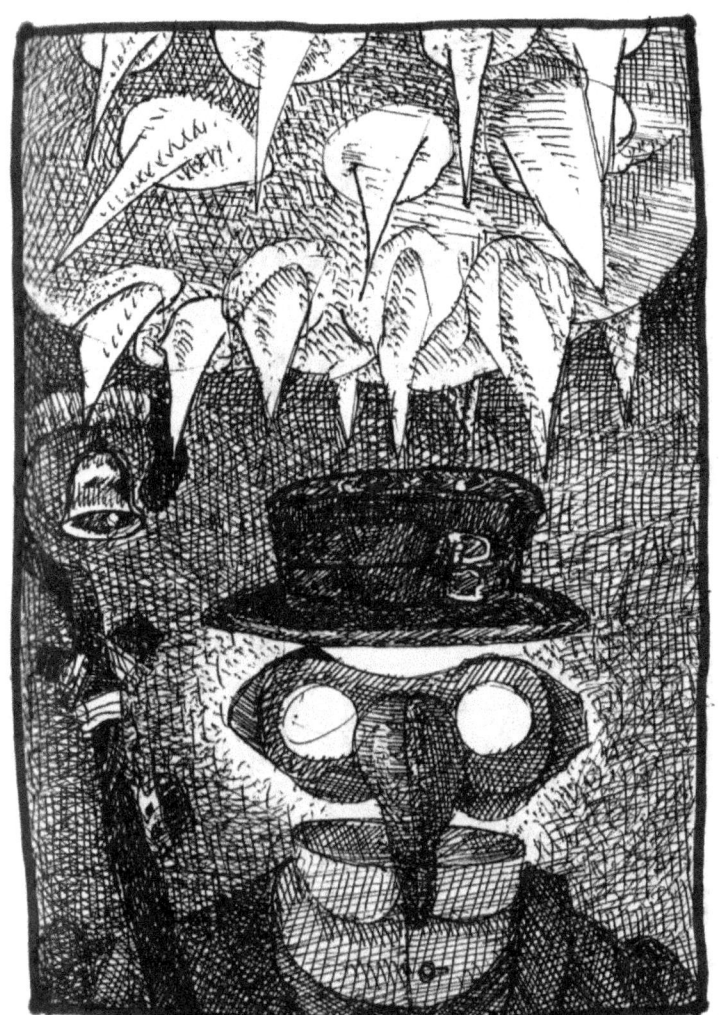

"Beneath the Belly of the Blast"

Mitchell

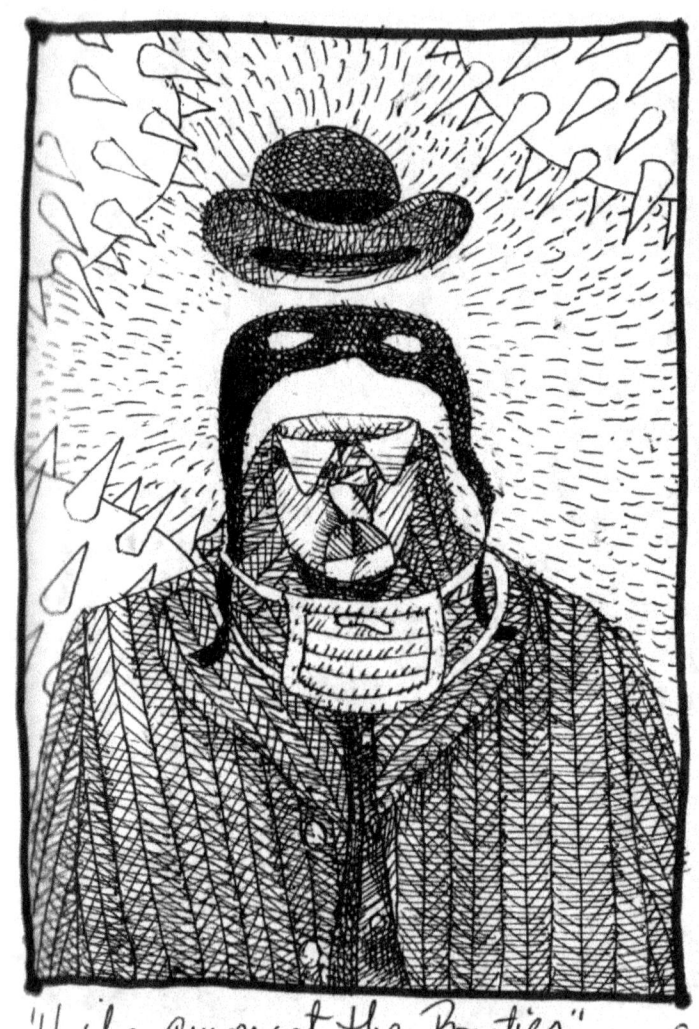

"Life amongst the Beasties"
Mitchell

March 31

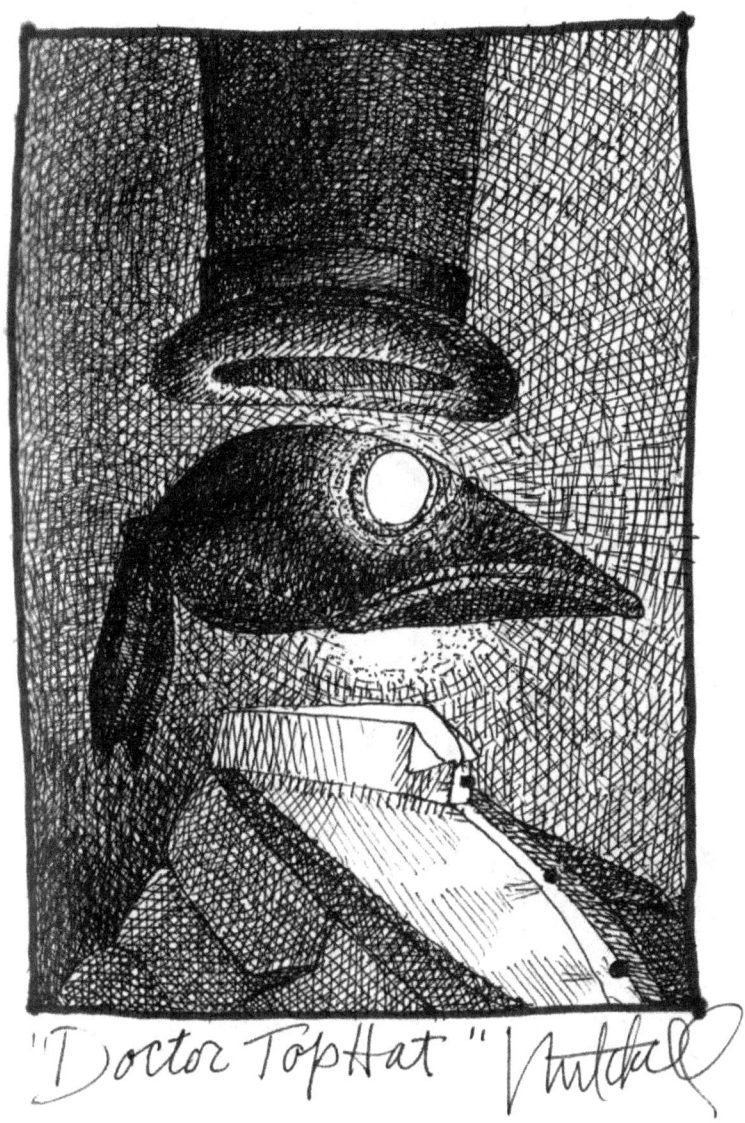

"Doctor TopHat"

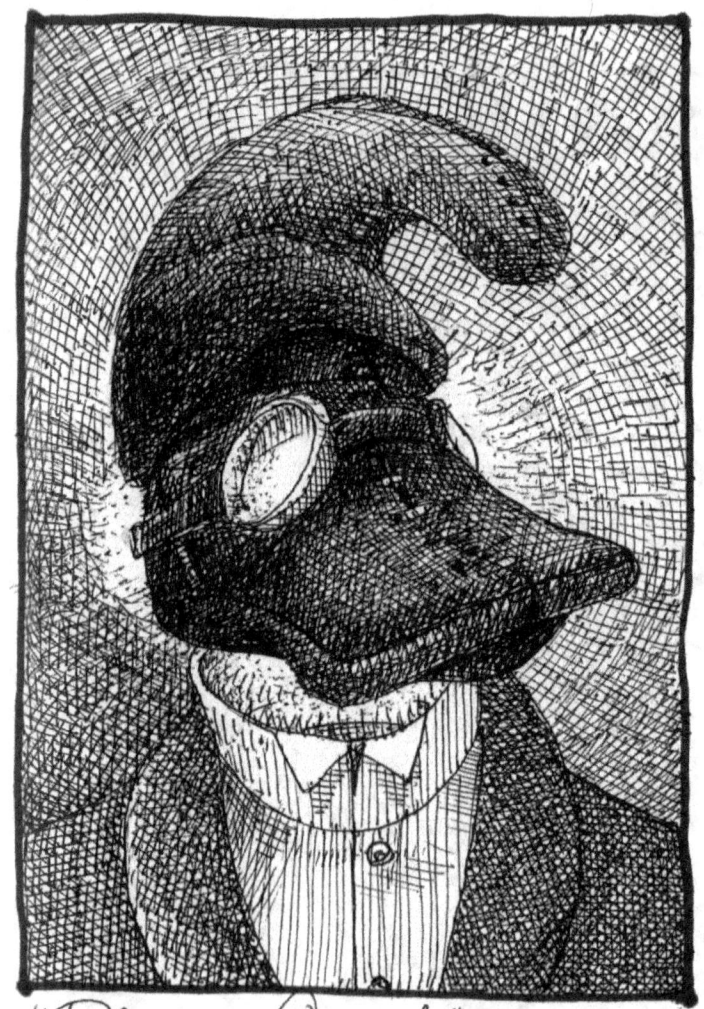

"Plague Quack" Mitchell

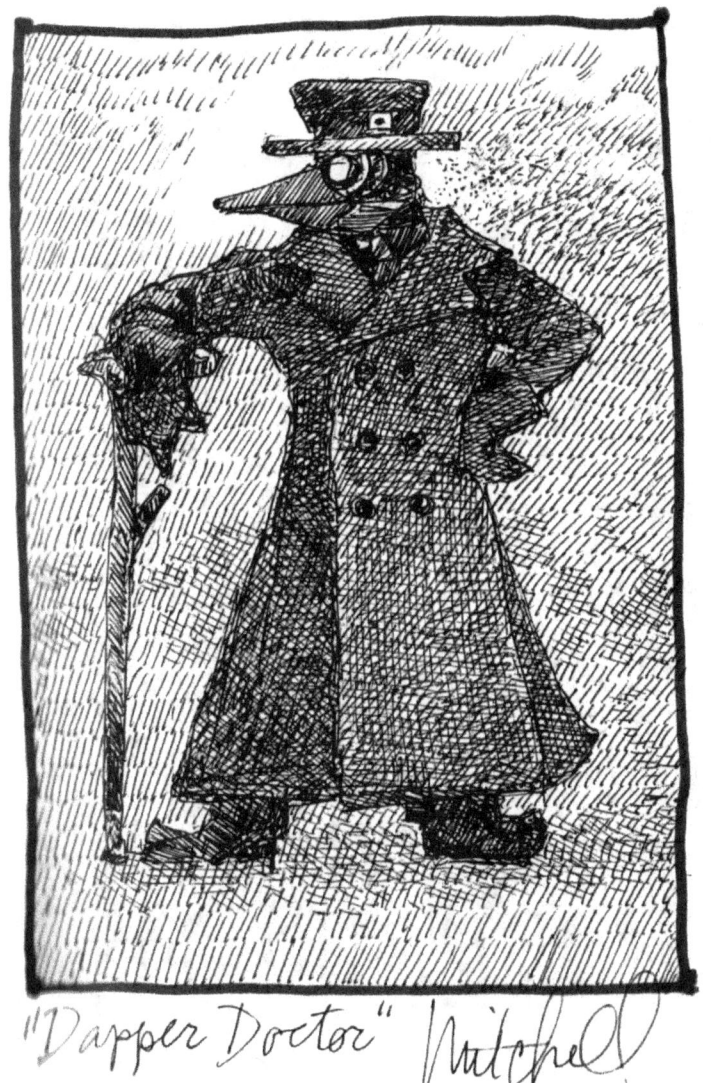

"Dapper Doctor" Mitchell

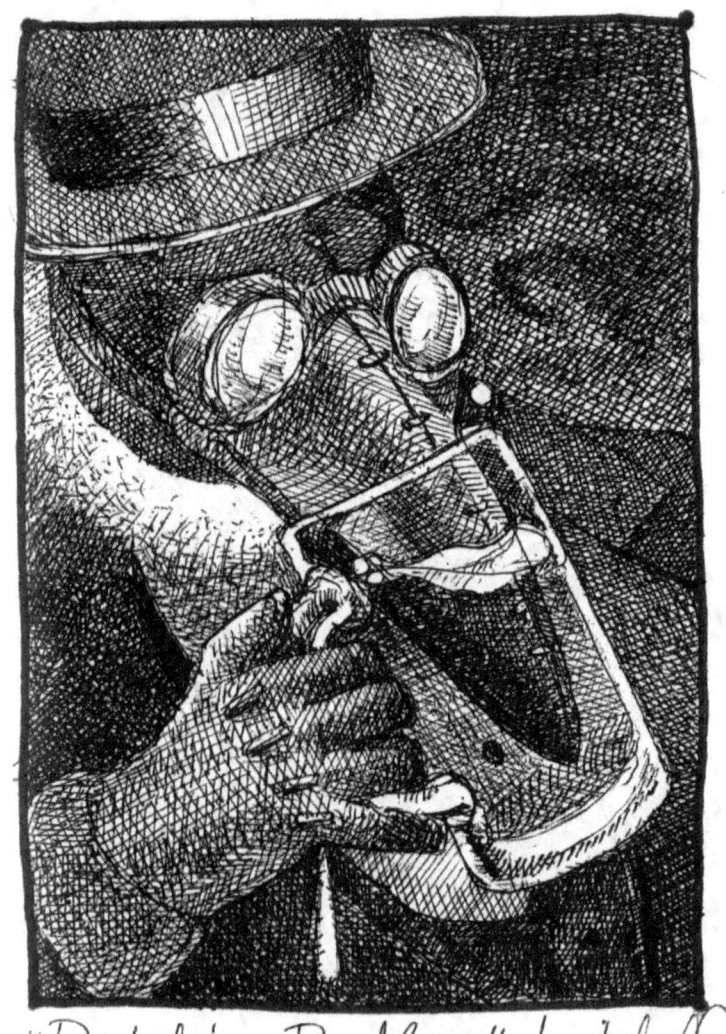

"Drinking Problem" Mitchell

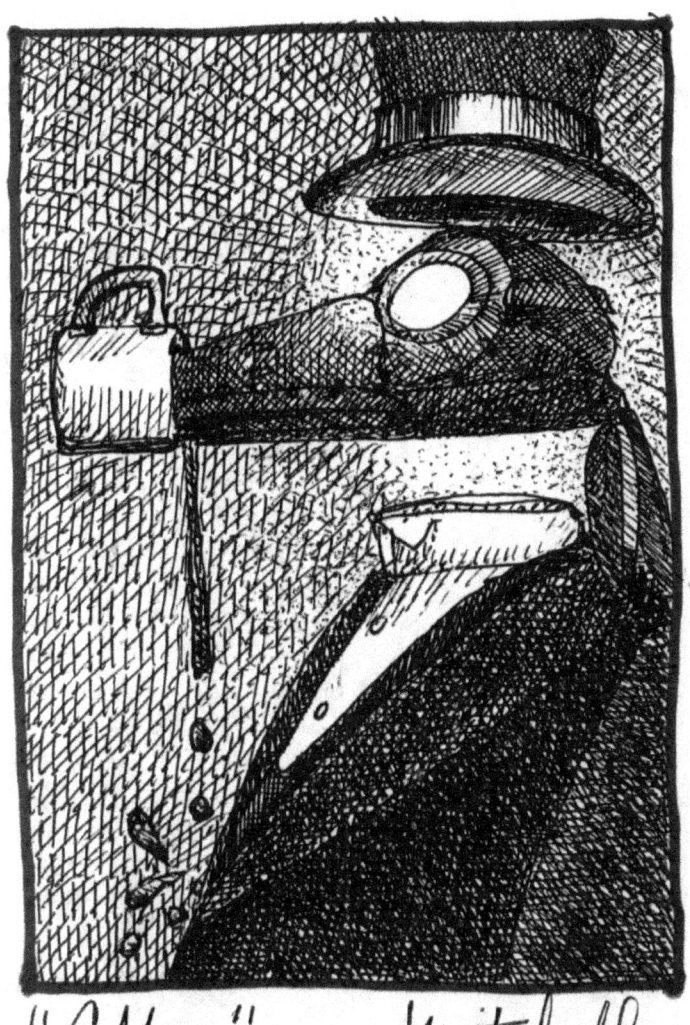

"*Coffee*" *Mitchell*

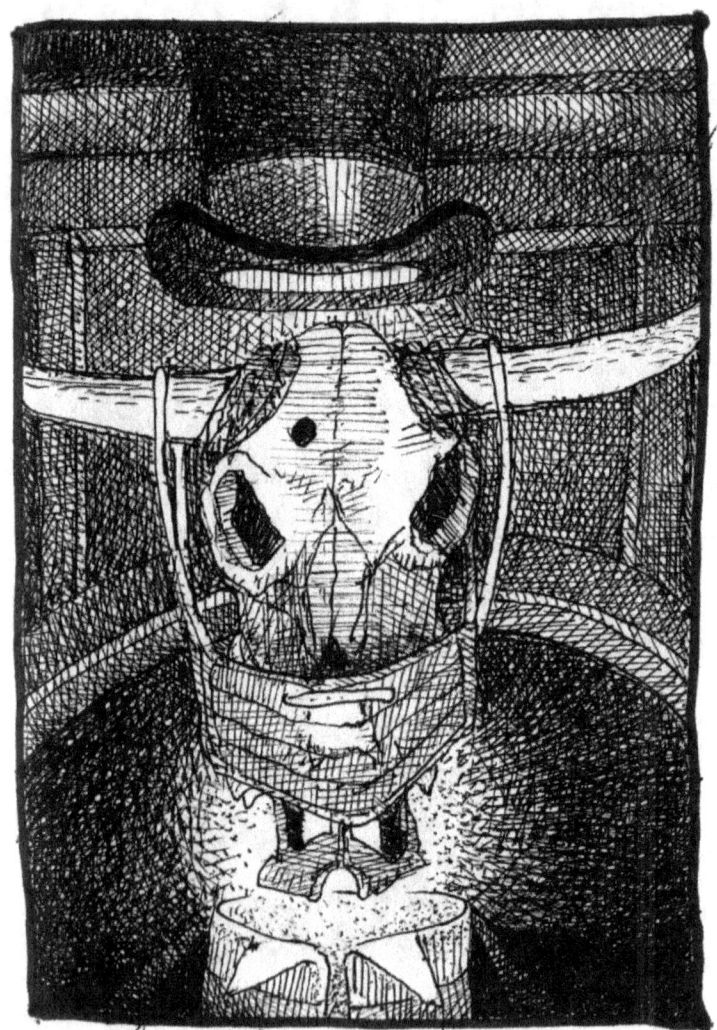

"Cowskull Bill Masks Up"

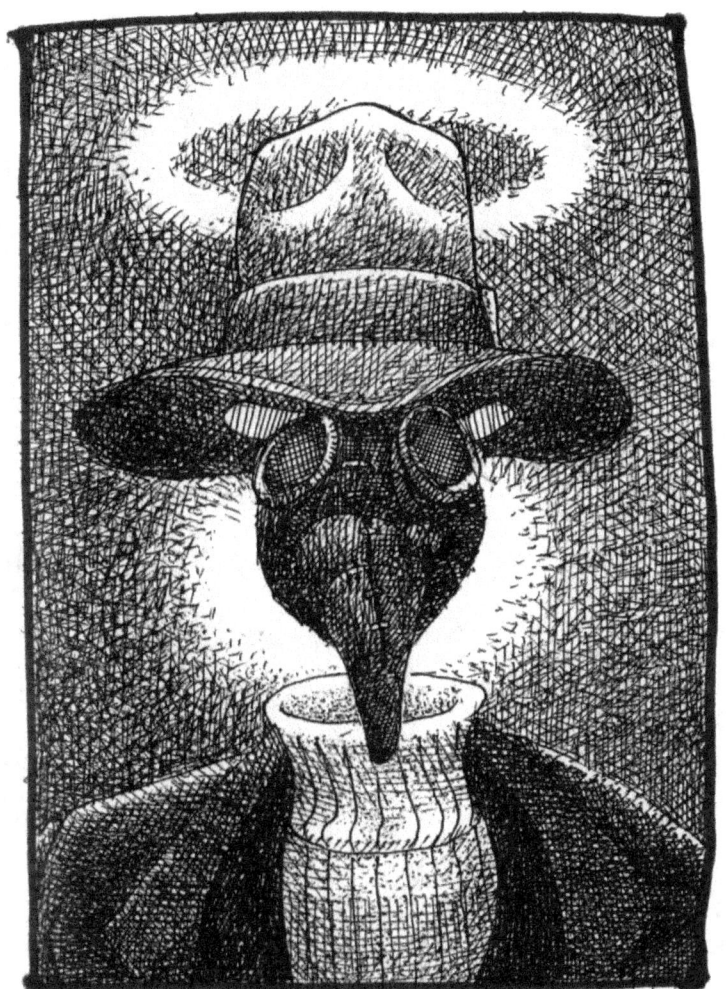

"Blessed Are the Plague Doctors"

Mitchell

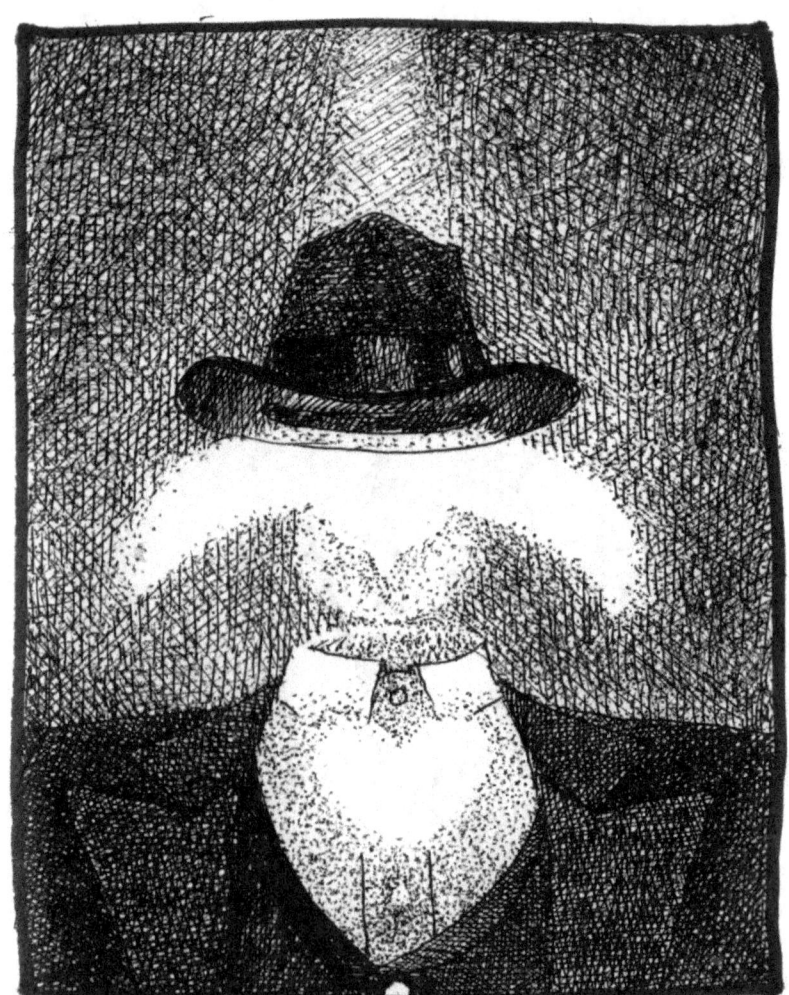

"Source of Compassion" Mitchell

April 7

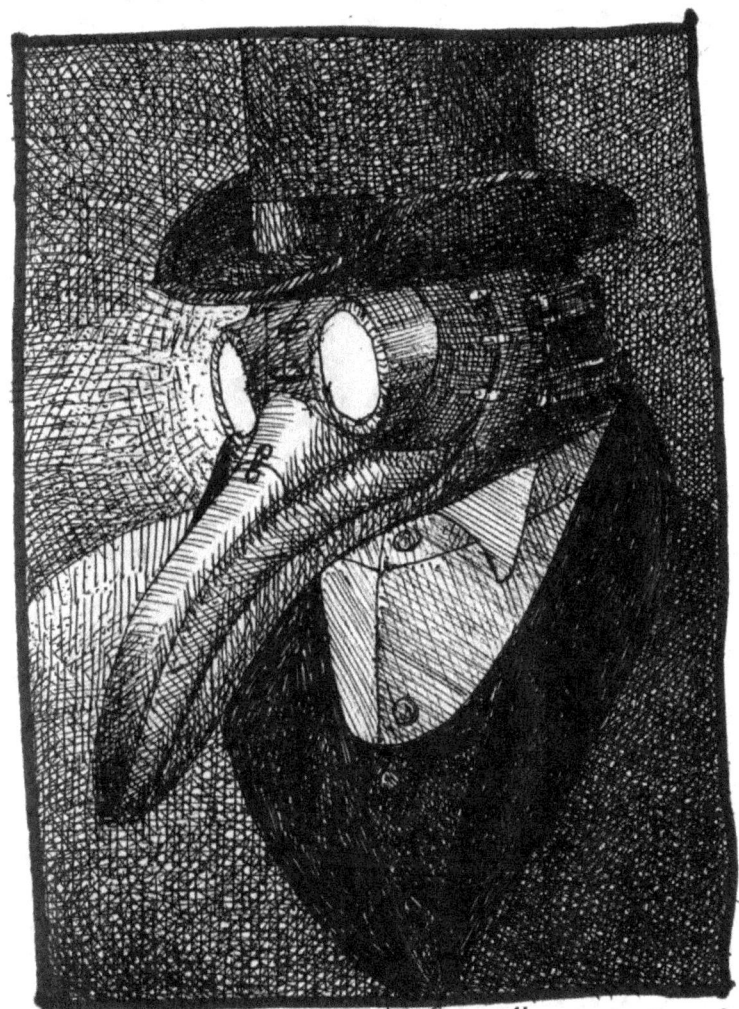

"the Light in Your Eyes" Mitchell

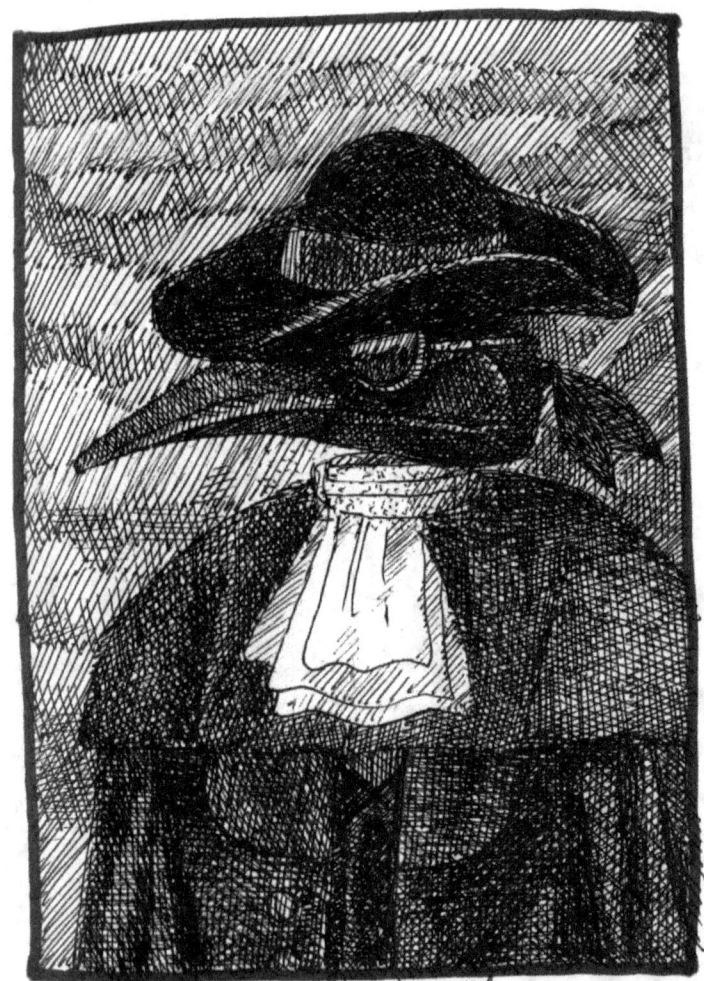

"Plague Doctor as Highwayman"

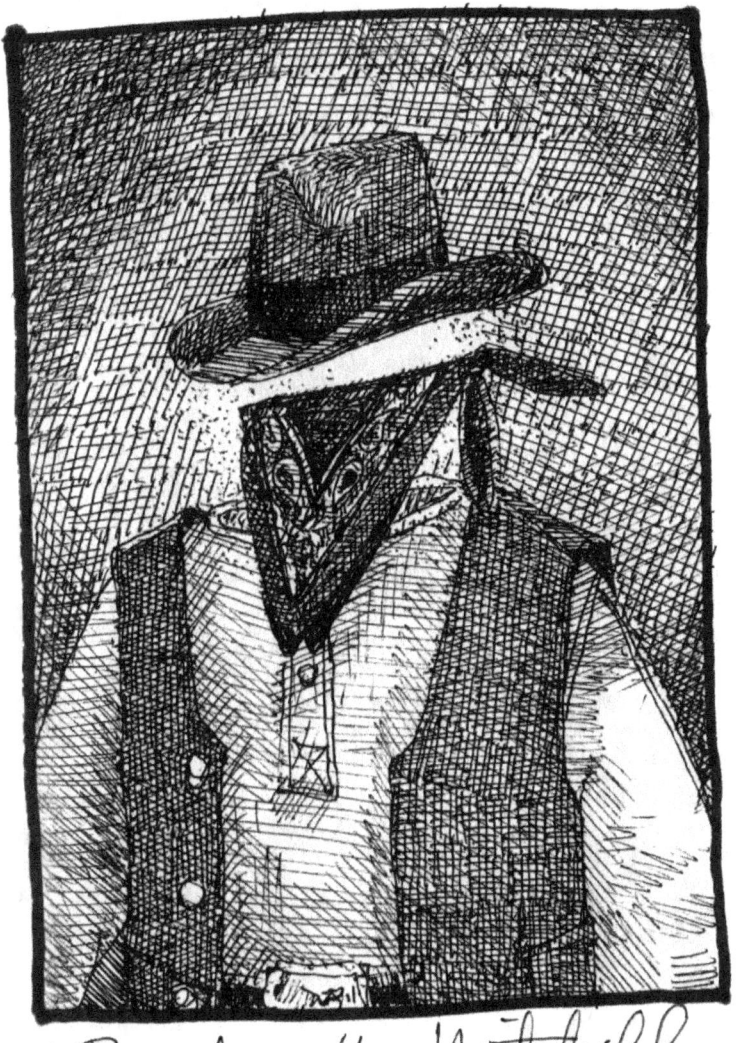

"Bandana" Mitchell

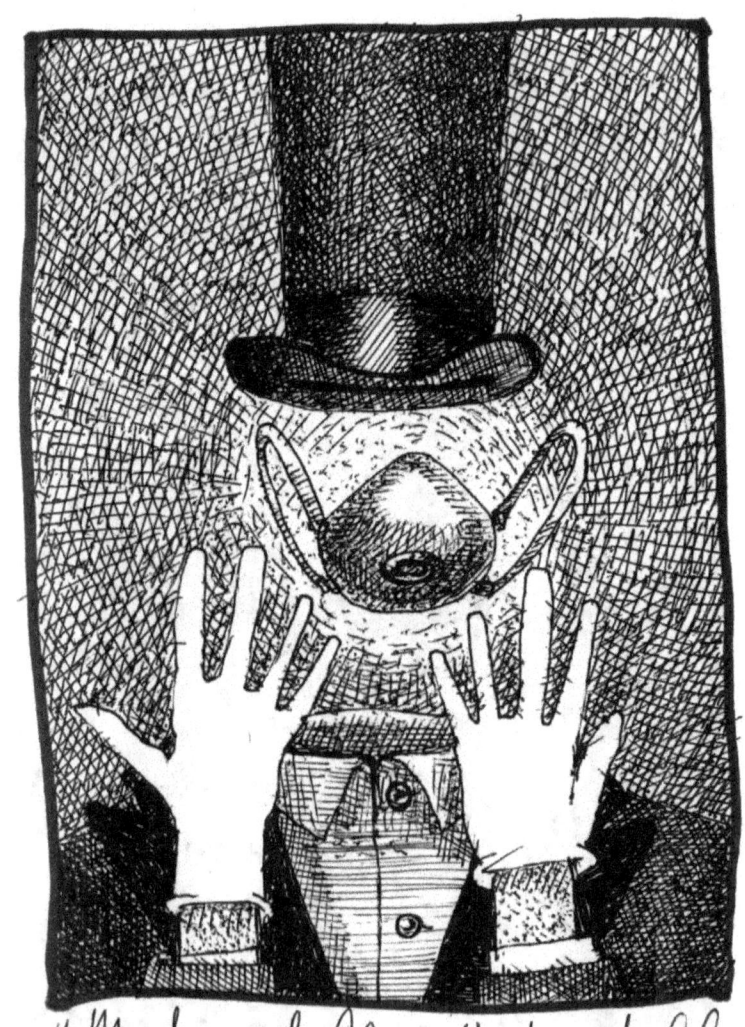

"Mask and Gloves" *Mitchell*

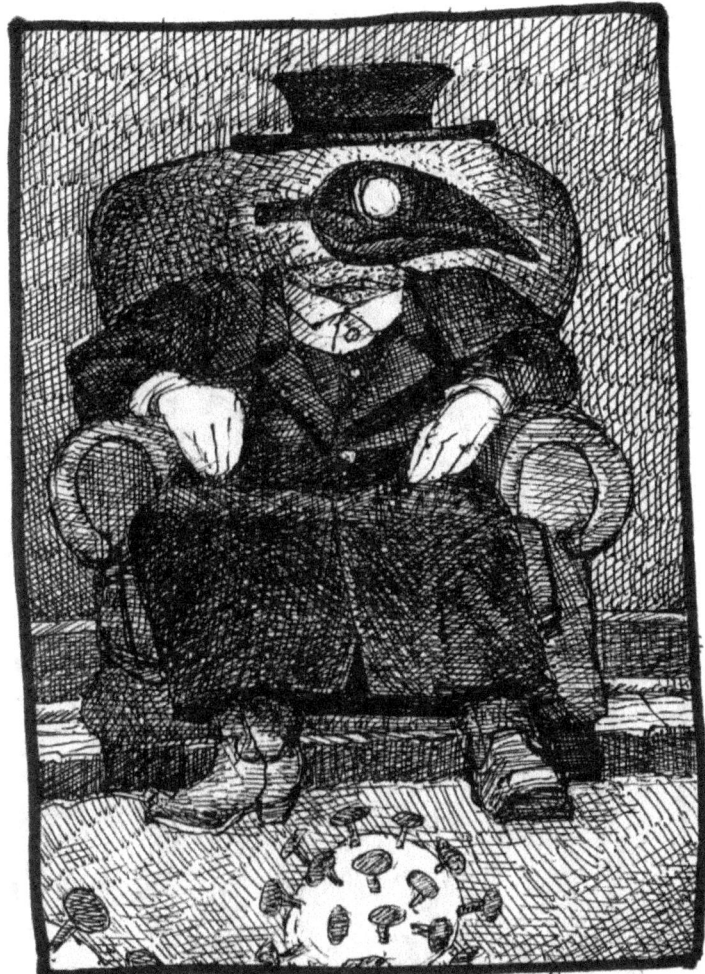

"Plague Doctor, Comfy Chair"
Mitchell

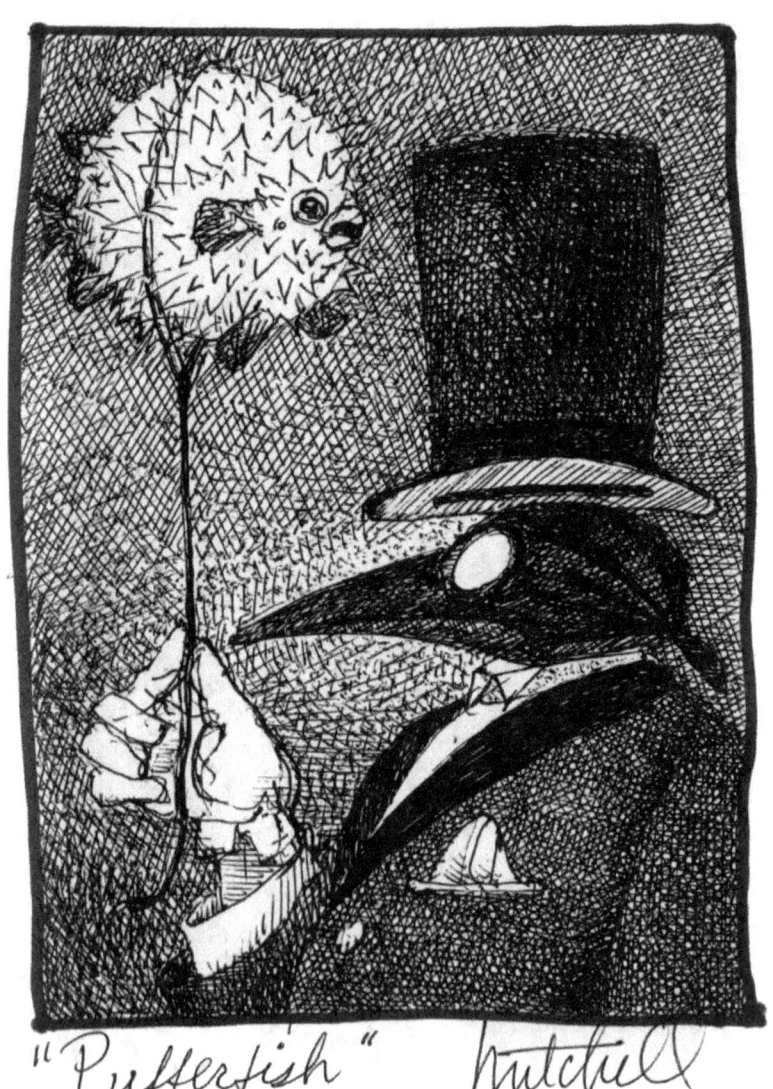

"Pufferfish"   Mitchell

April 13

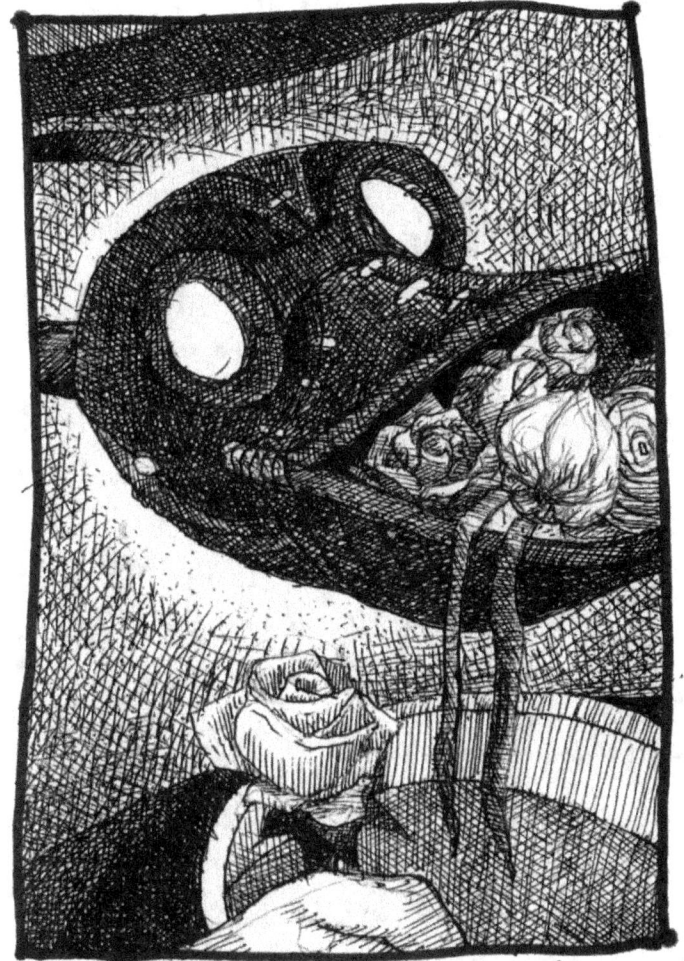

"Repleneshing the Essentials"
Roses and Garlic

Mitchell

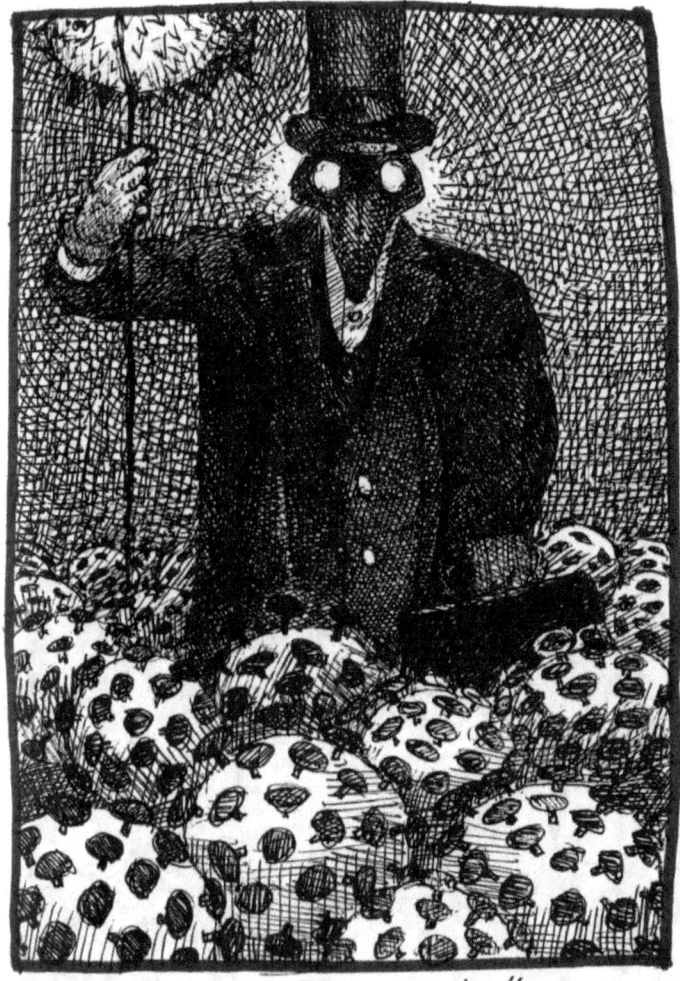

"Knee-deep in Pandemia"

Mitchull

April 18

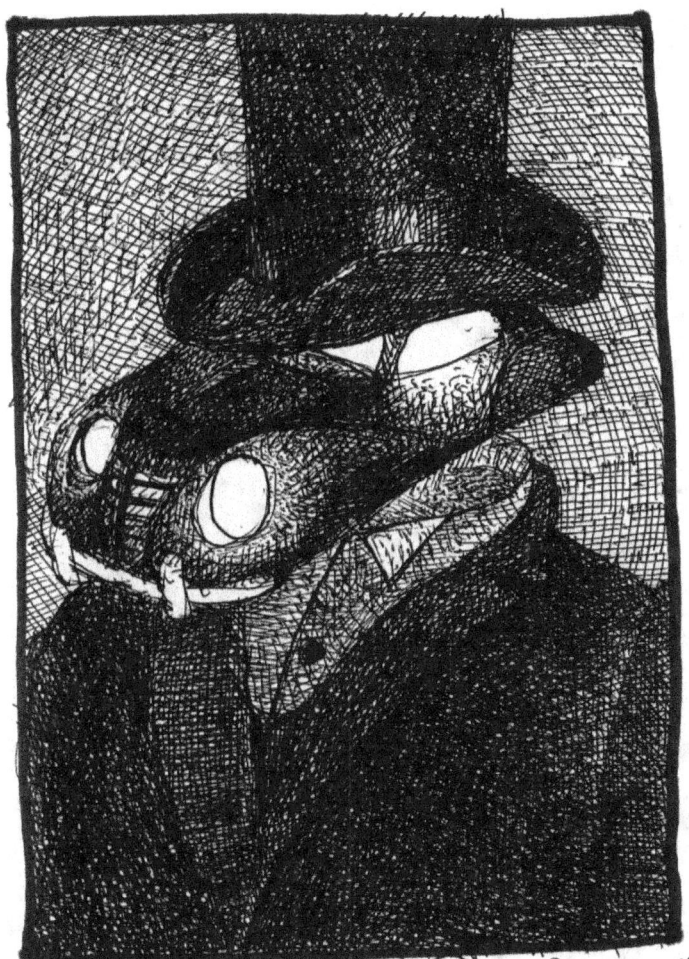

"Plague Doctor as Deco Coupe"
Mitchell

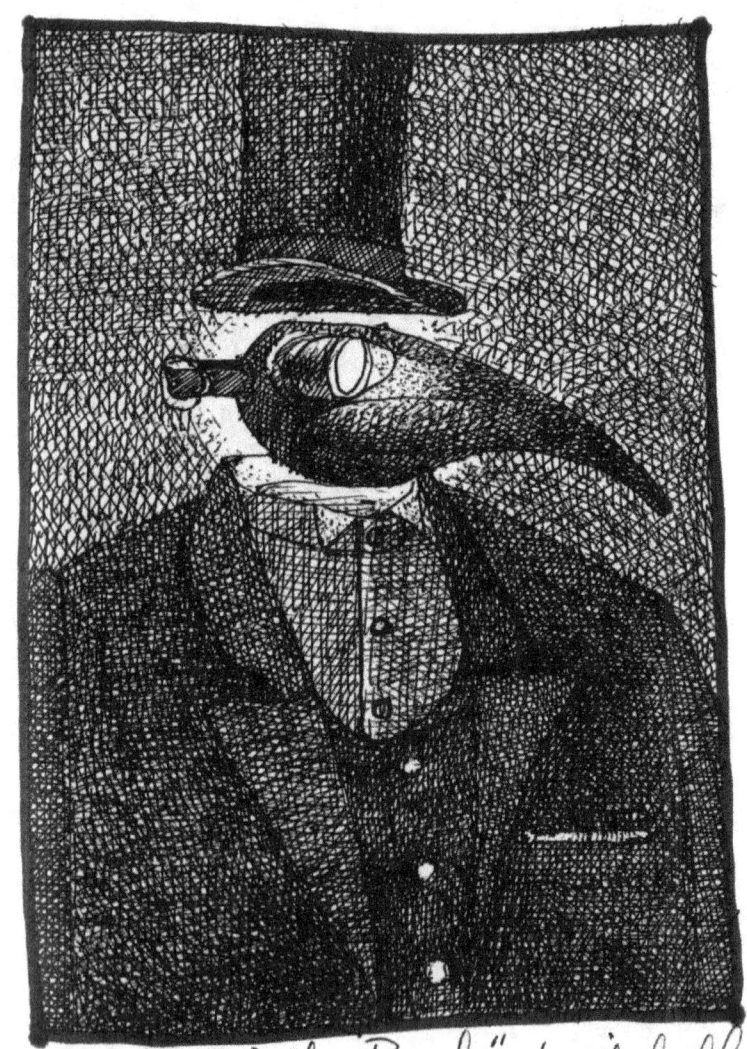

"Buckled in the Back" Mitchull

April 22

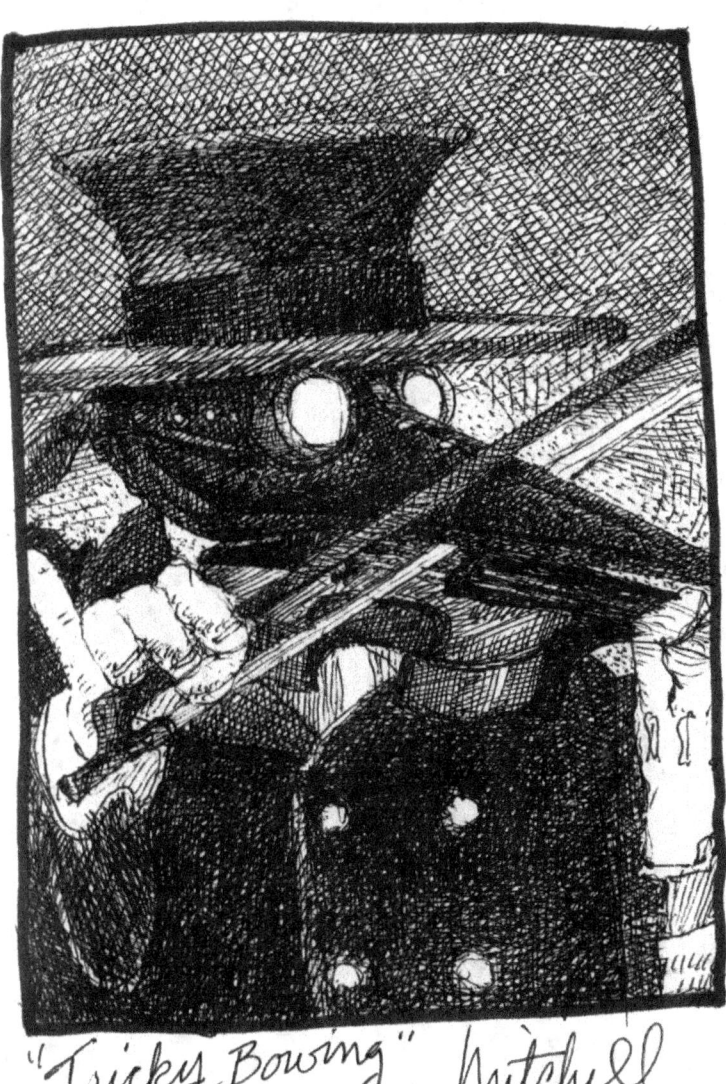

"Tricky Bowing" Mitchell

April 24

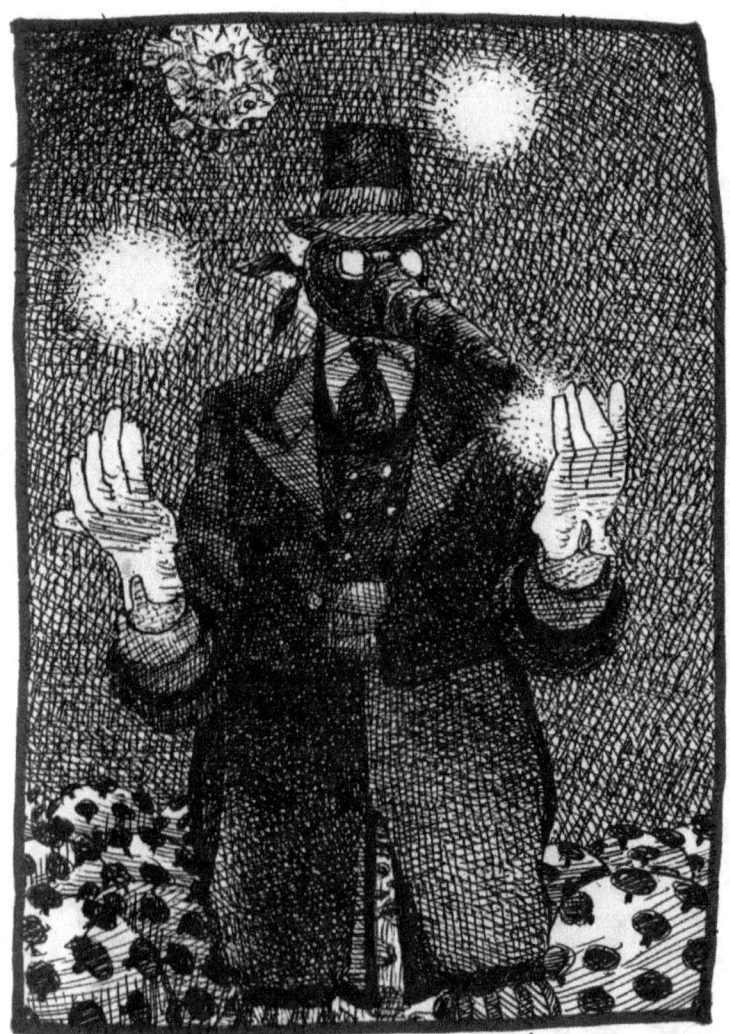

"The Master Juggler" Mitchell

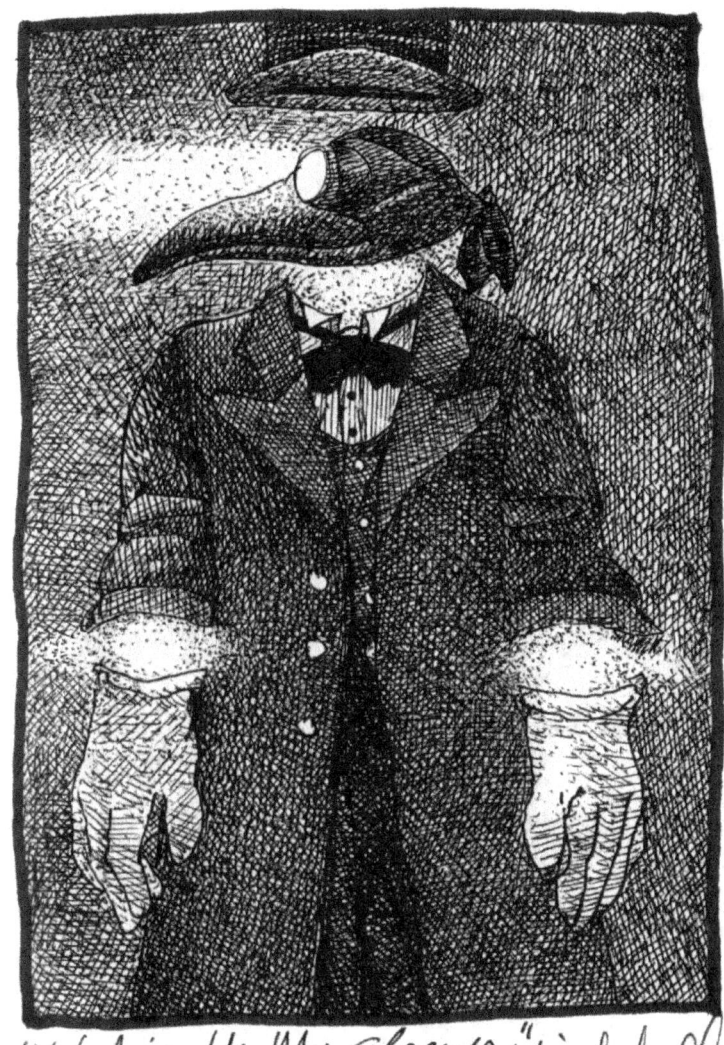

"Nothing Up My Sleeves" *Mitchell*

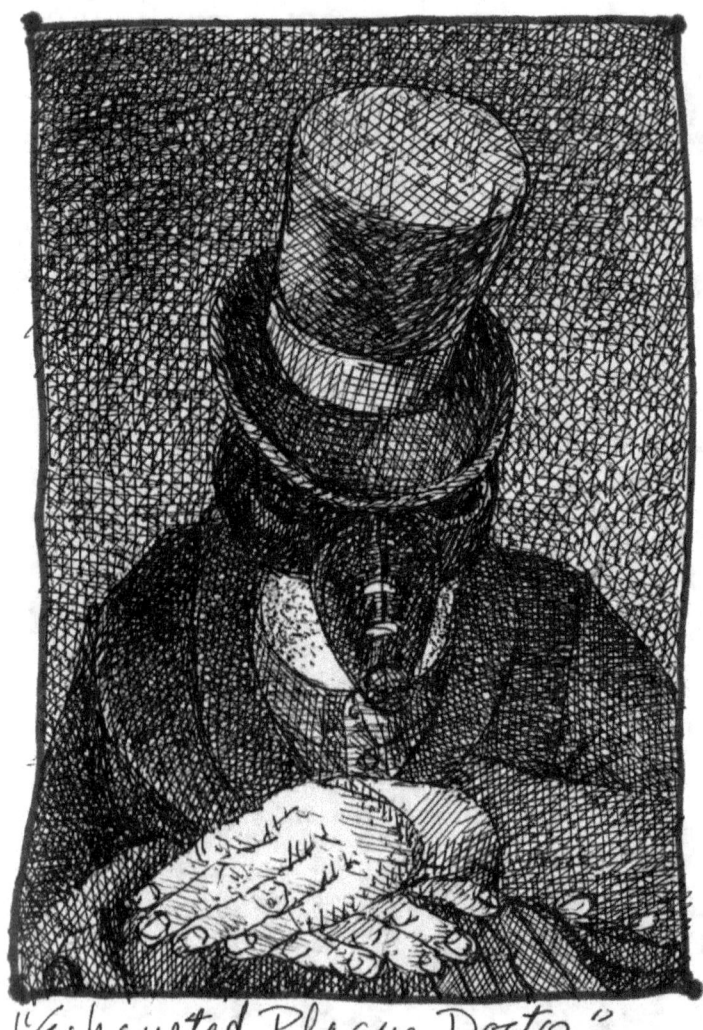

"Exhausted Plague Doctor"
Mitchell

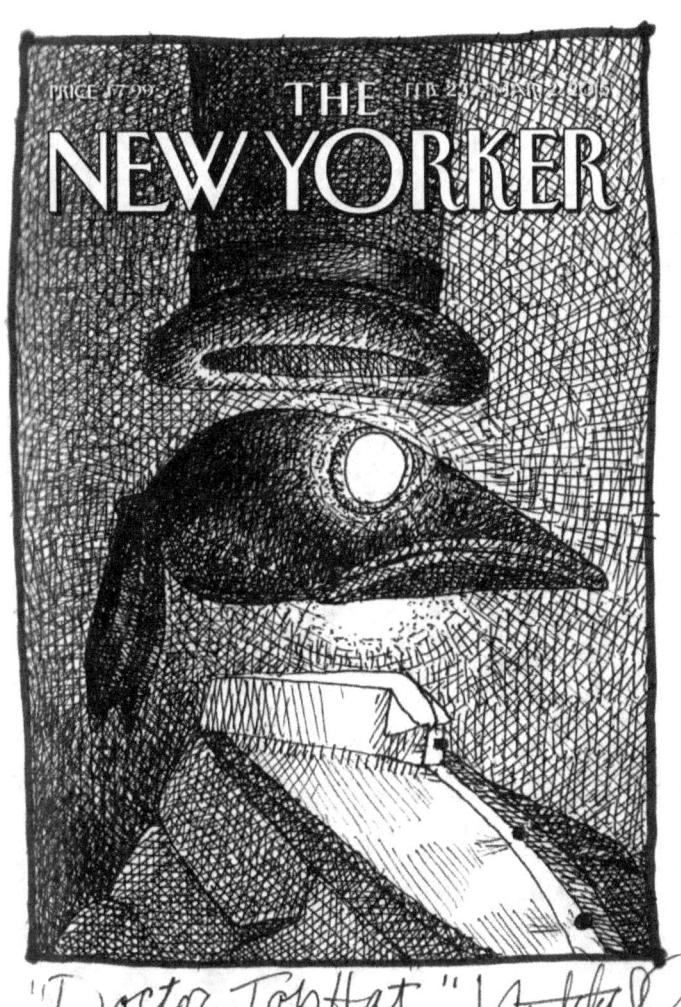

"Doctor TopHat"

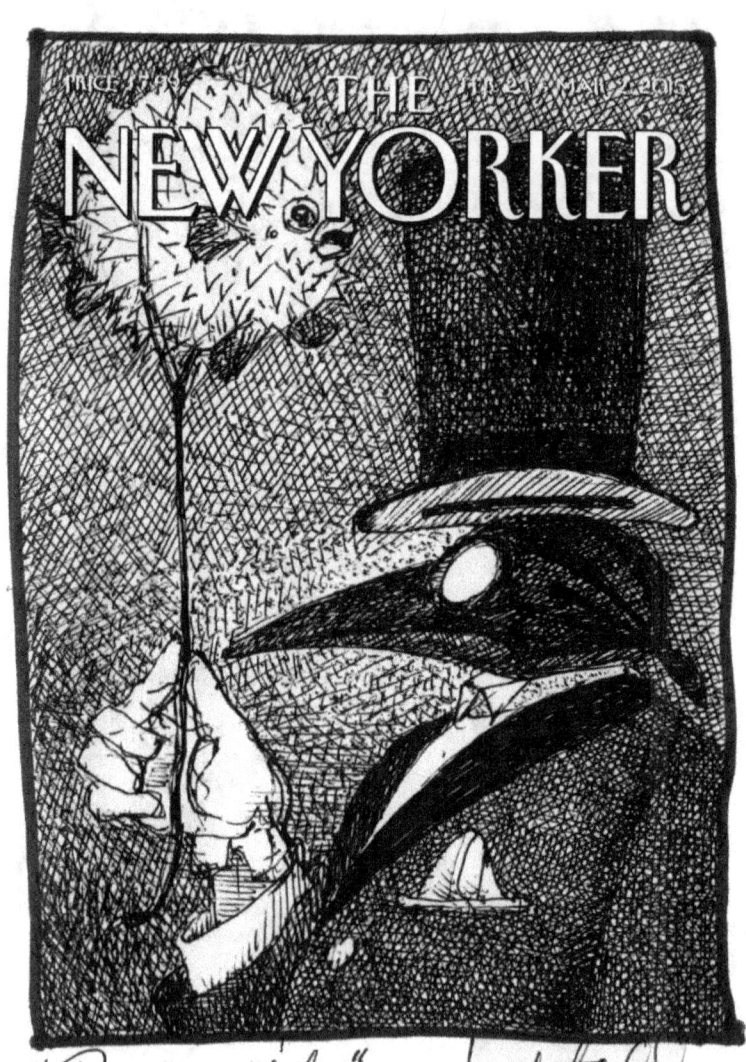

"Pufferfish"   Mitchell

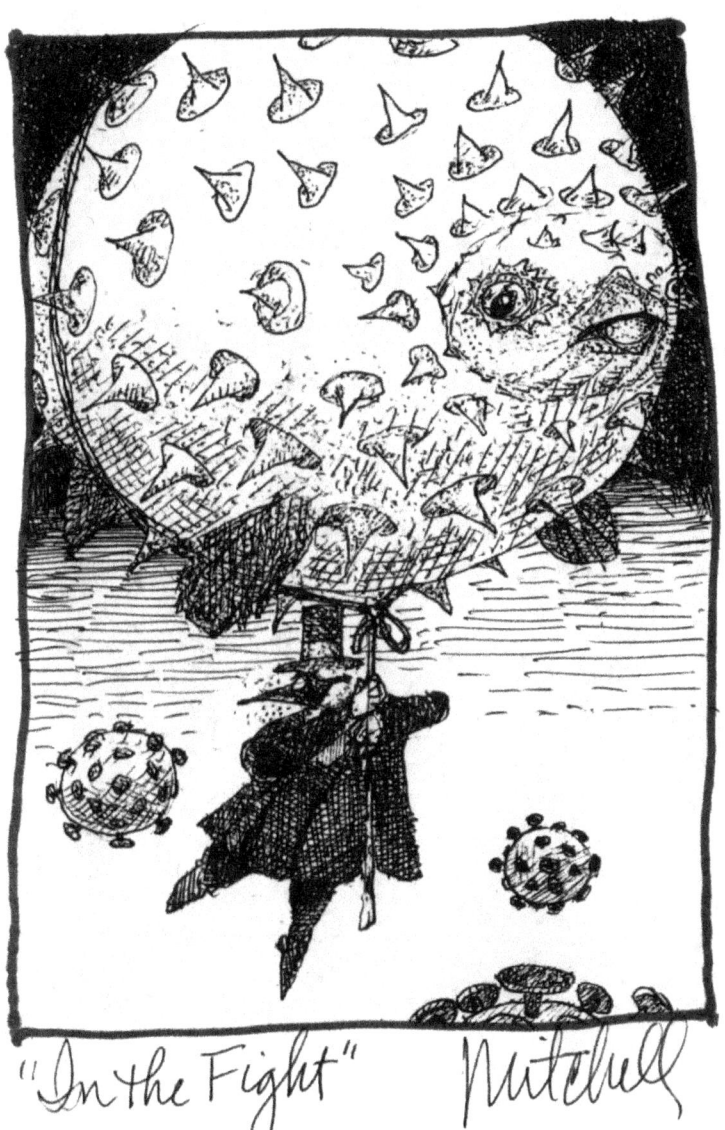

"In the Fight"   Mitchell

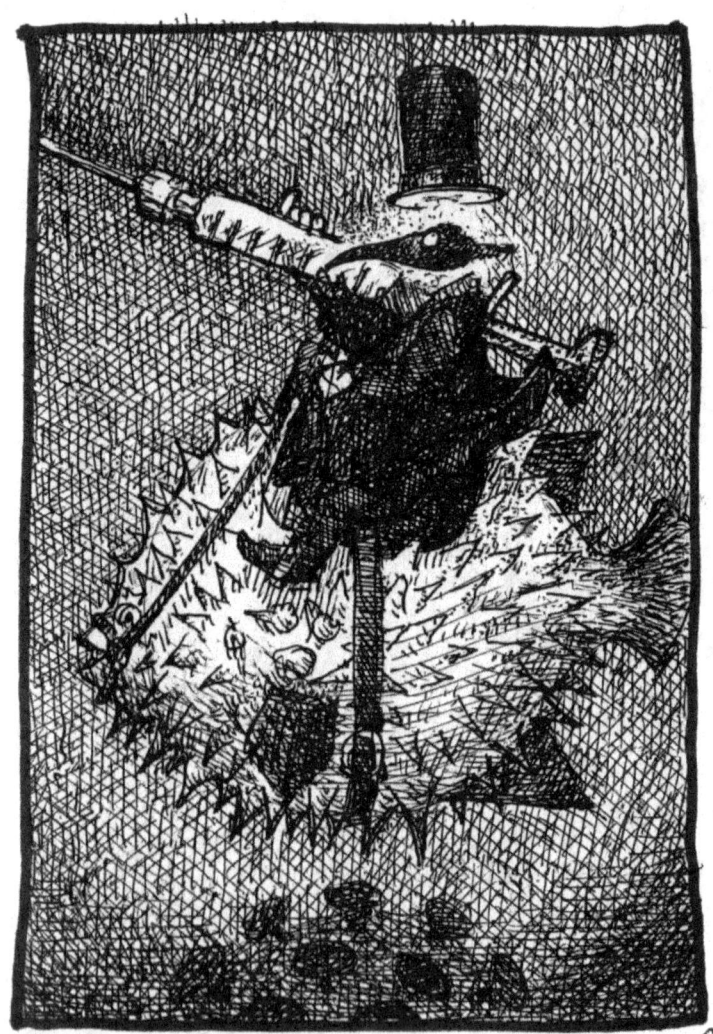

"Riding into Battle" Mitchell

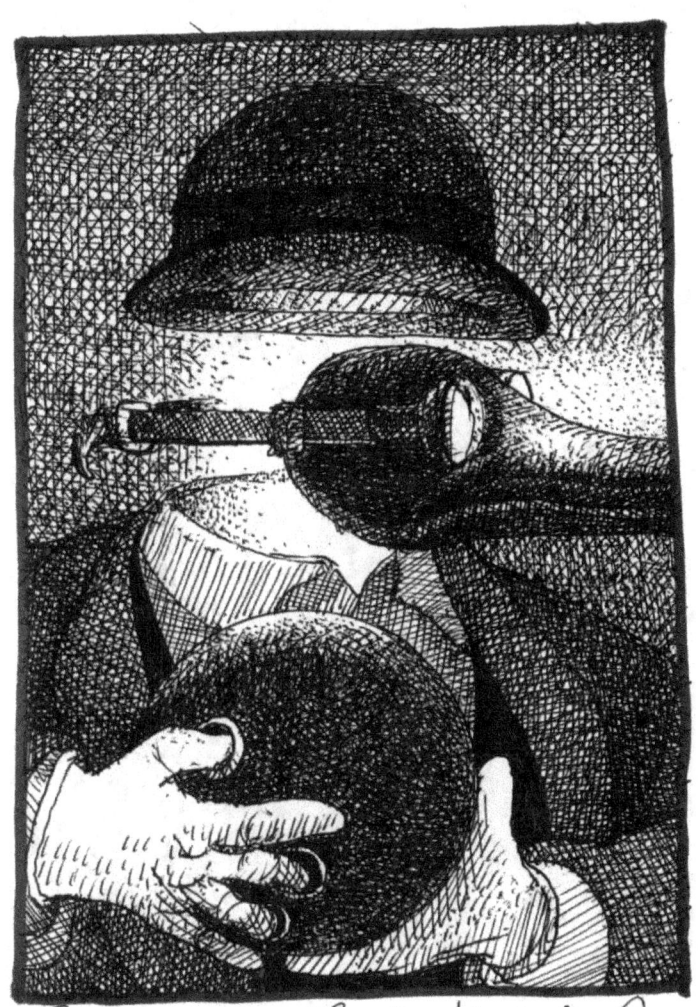

"Bowler Bowler"

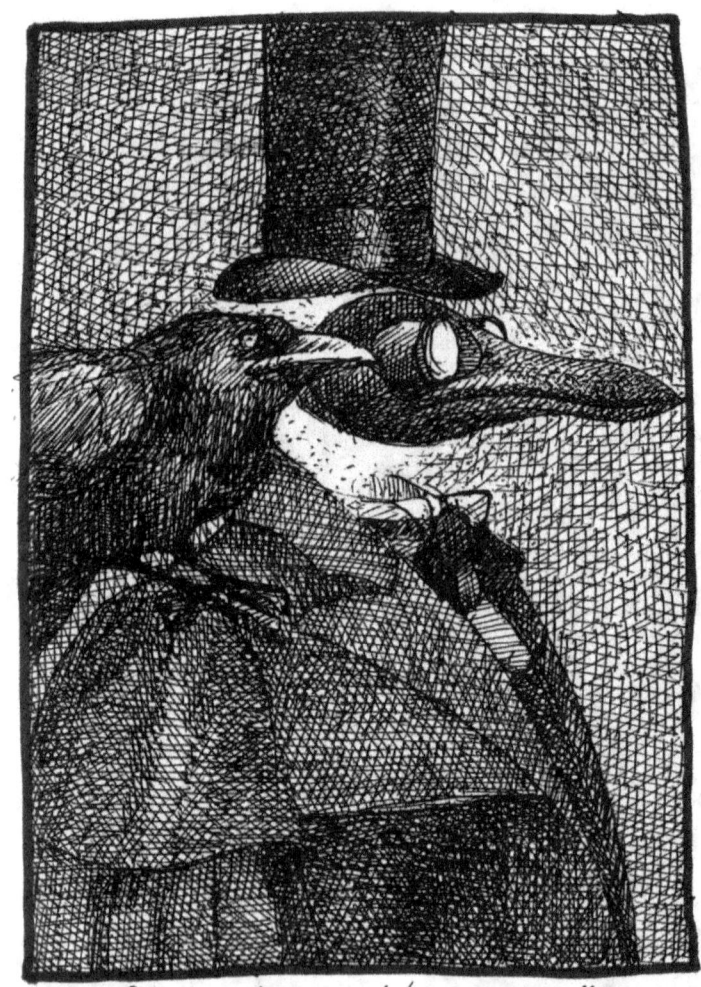

"World Pandemic, Nevermore"

Mitchell

May 4

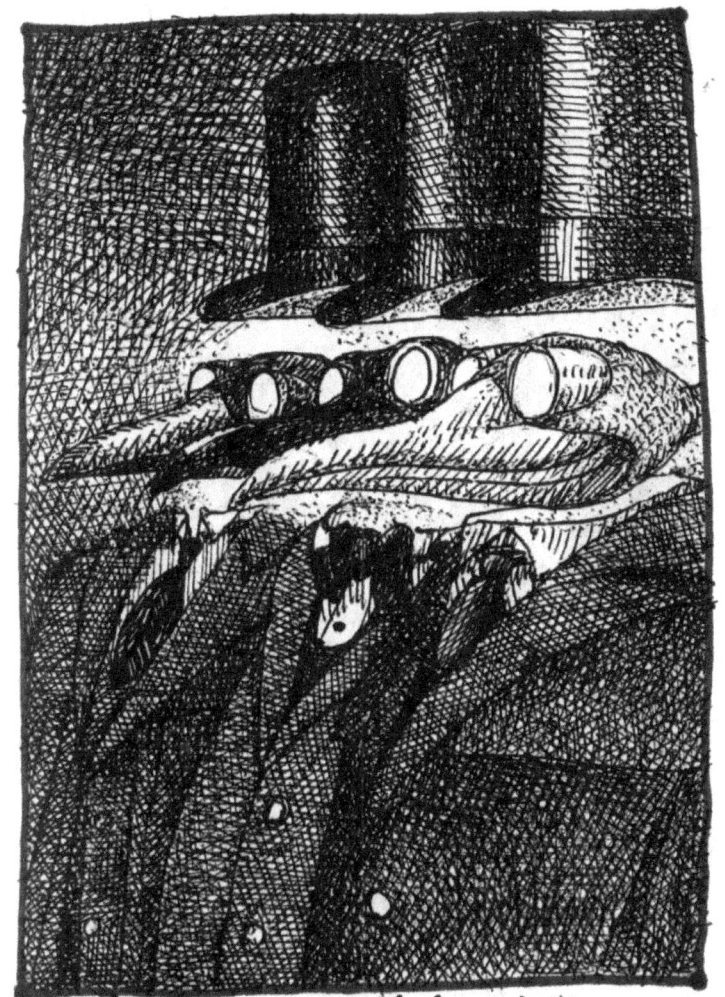

"All Cultures, All Creeds."

May 6

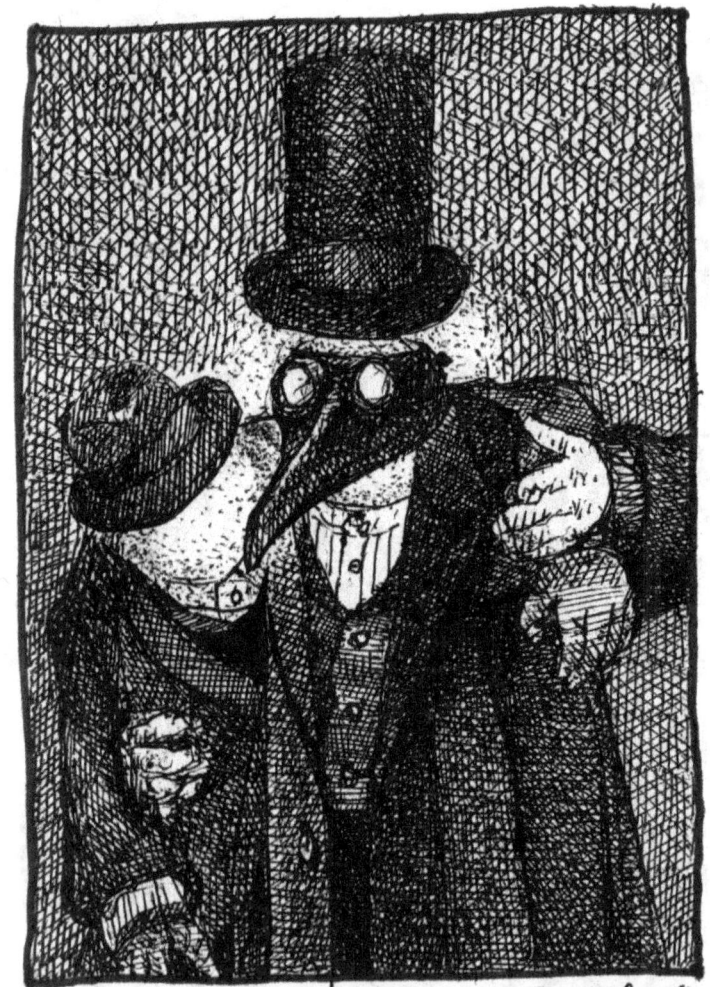

"He Ain't Heavy, He's My Brother"

Mitchell

May 8

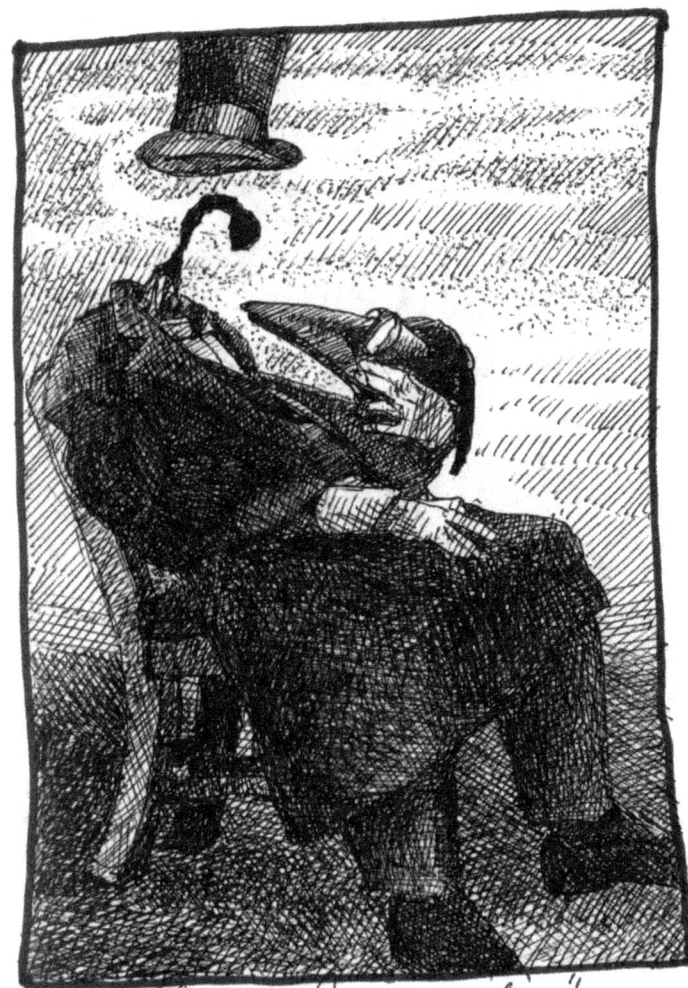

"Burned Out and Introspective"

Mitchell

May 9

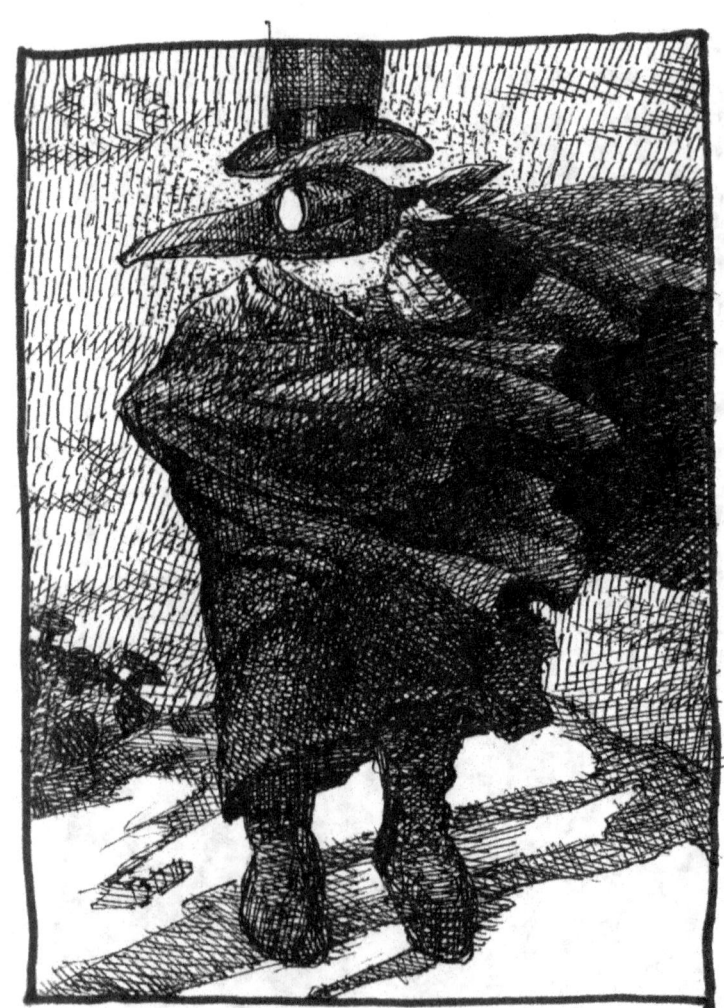

"Standing Against the Storm"

Mitchell

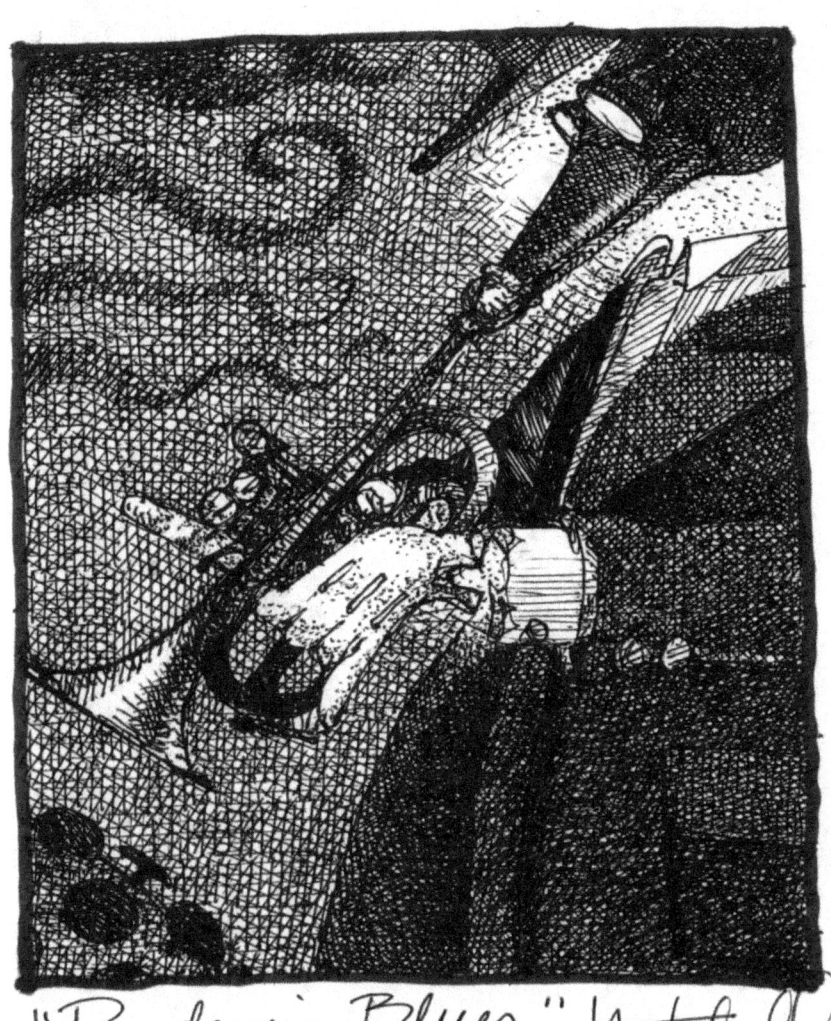

"*Pandemic Blues*" *Mitchell*

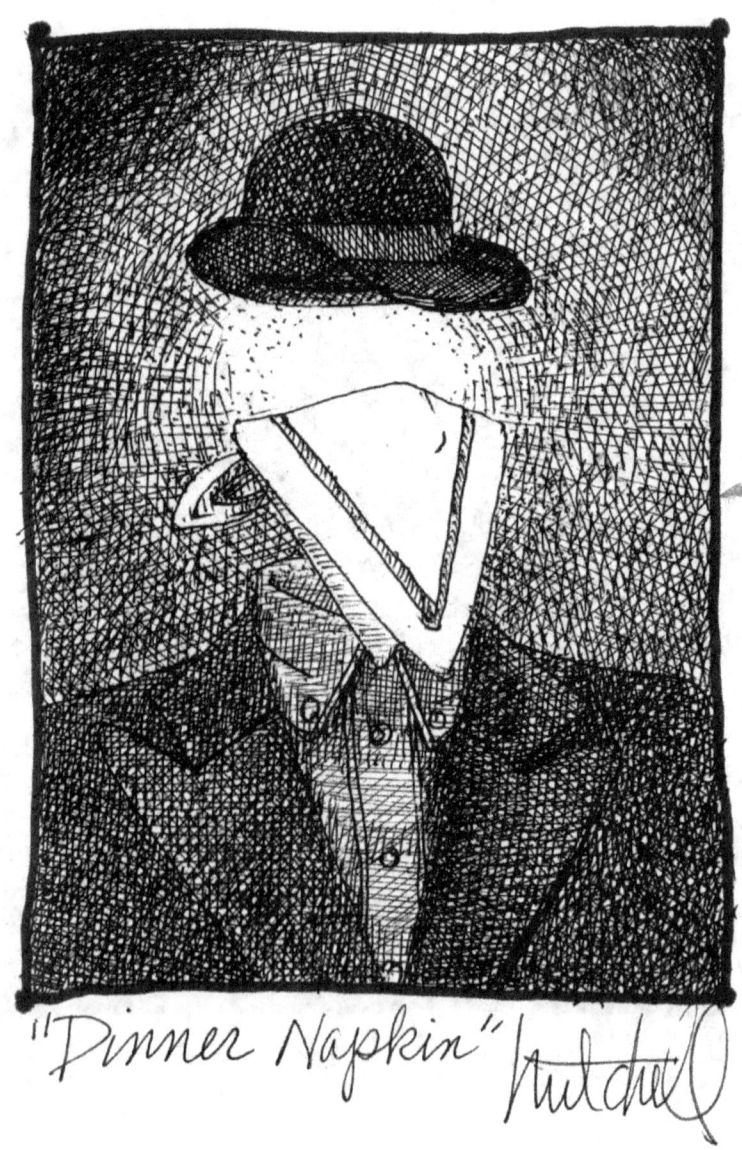

"Dinner Napkin"

May 14

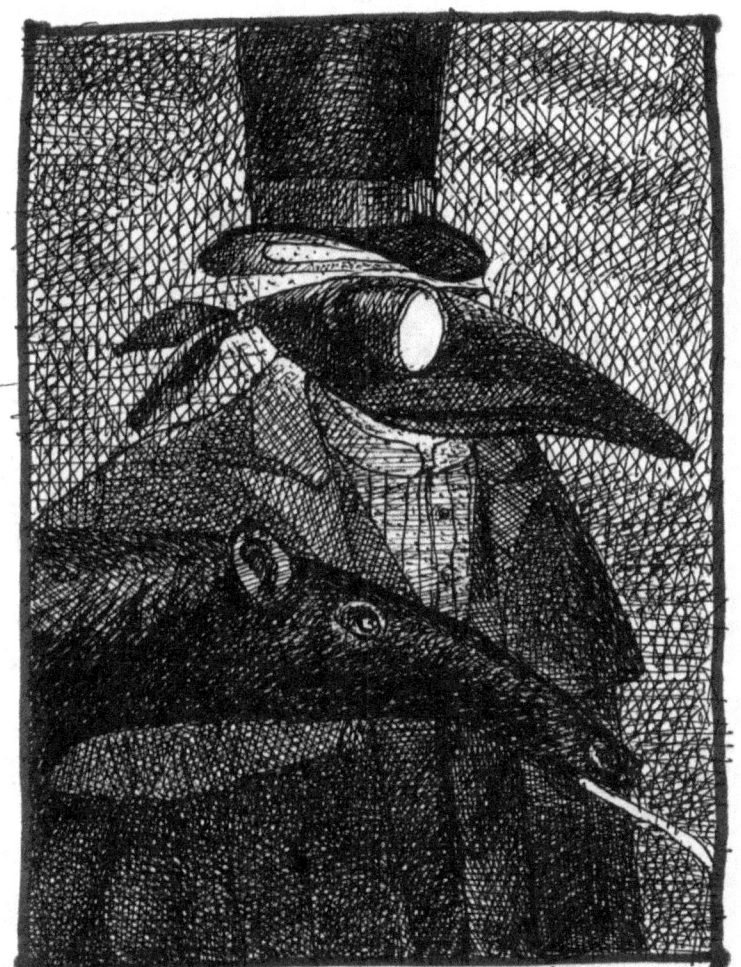

"Plague Doctor w/ anteater" mitchell

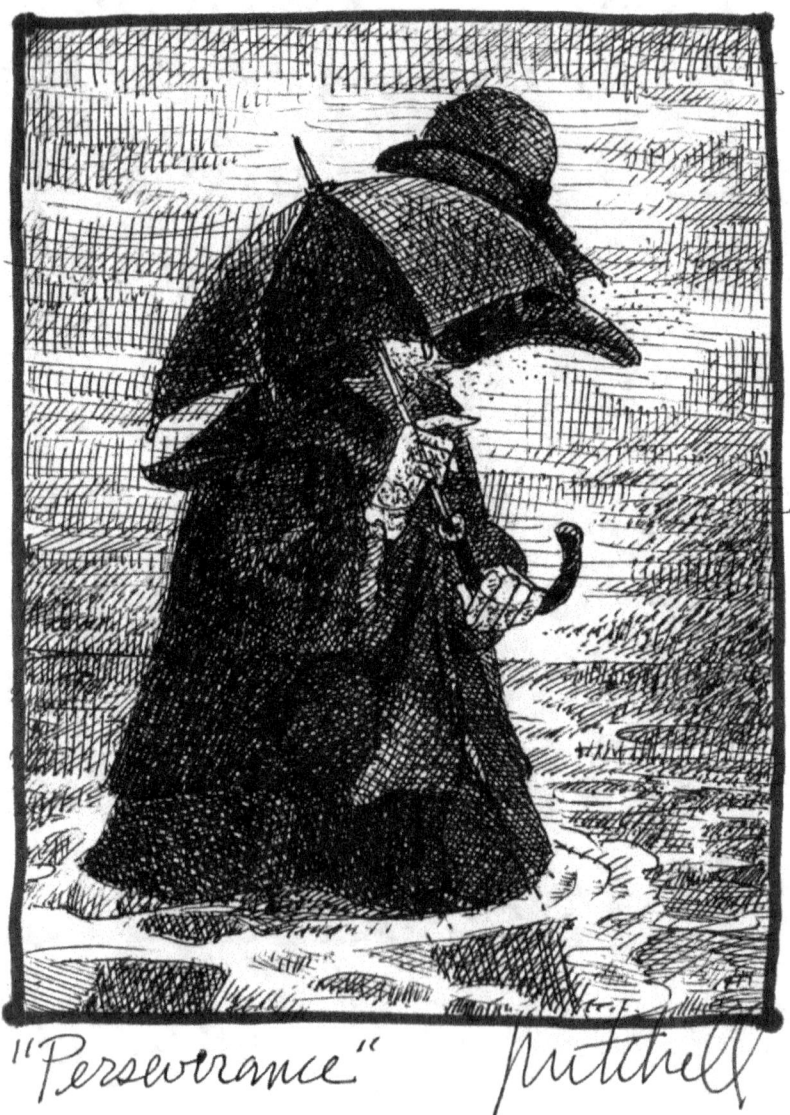

"*Perseverance*"

May 16

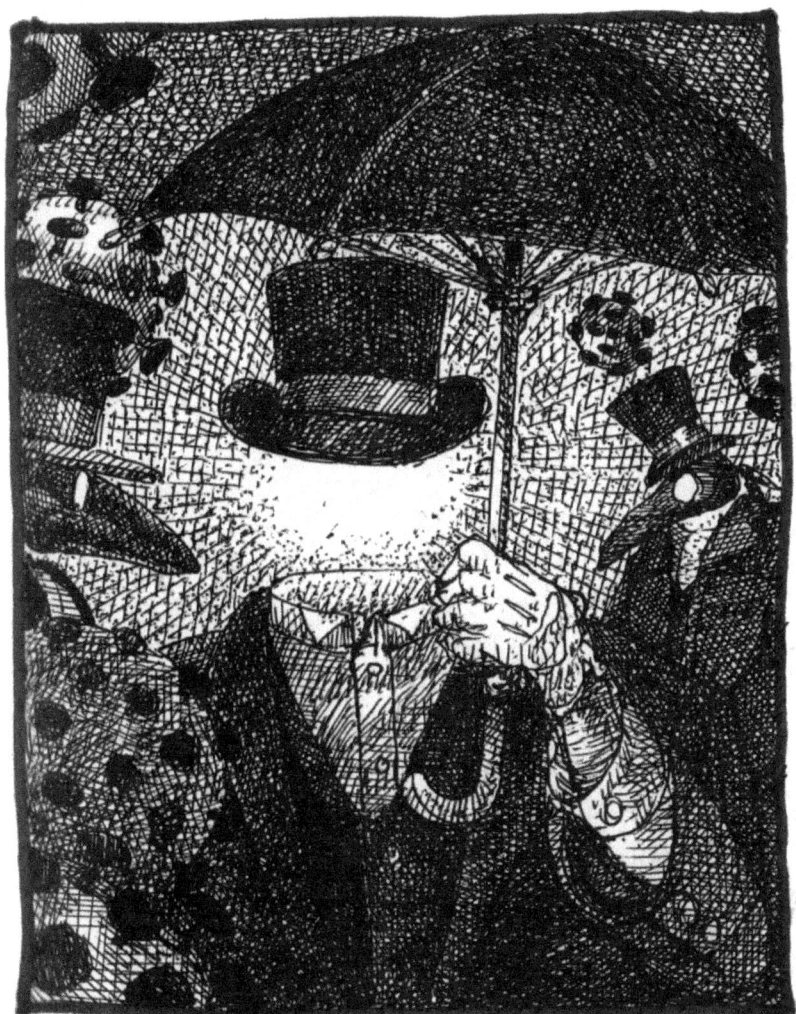

"Out Without a Mask" *Mitchell*

I had just finished this drawing this morning when I learned via text message that a young man I know from my church had just been released from a 10 day stay in the hospital due to Covid-19. He is a young athletic man ... it makes me take a look again at this treacherous virus. His father was also affected.—KM

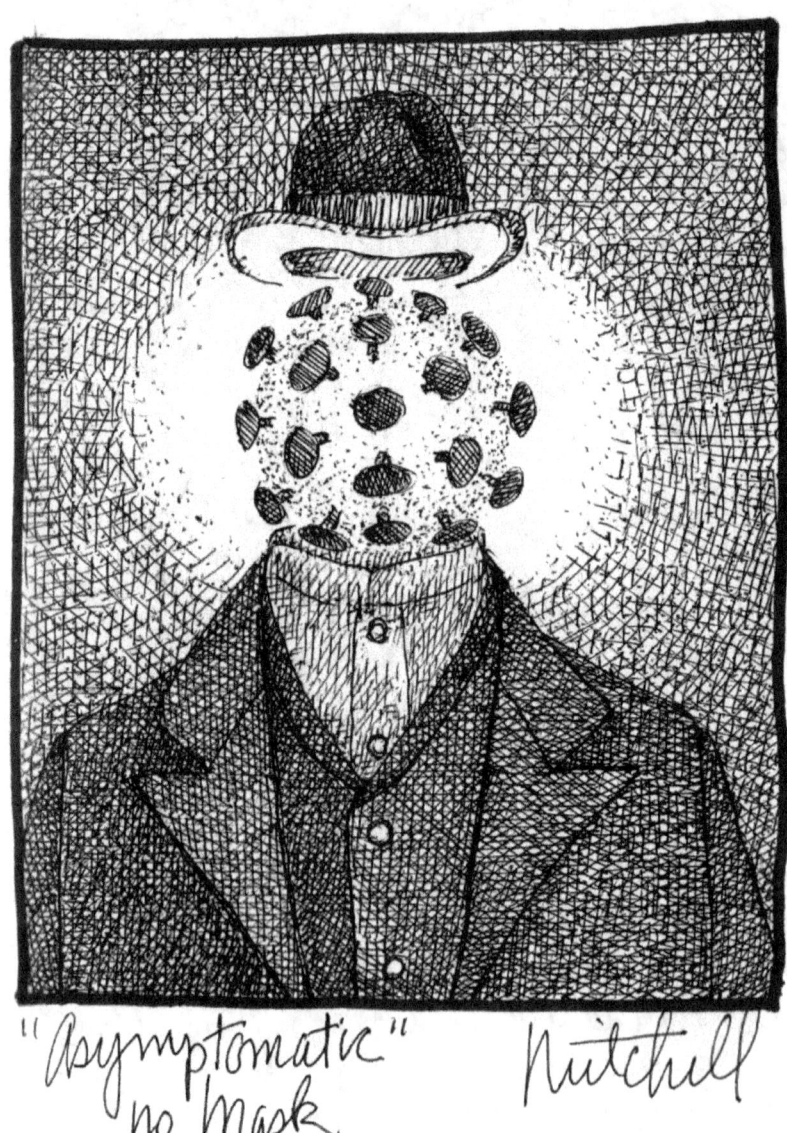

"Asymptomatic"
no Mask

Mitchell

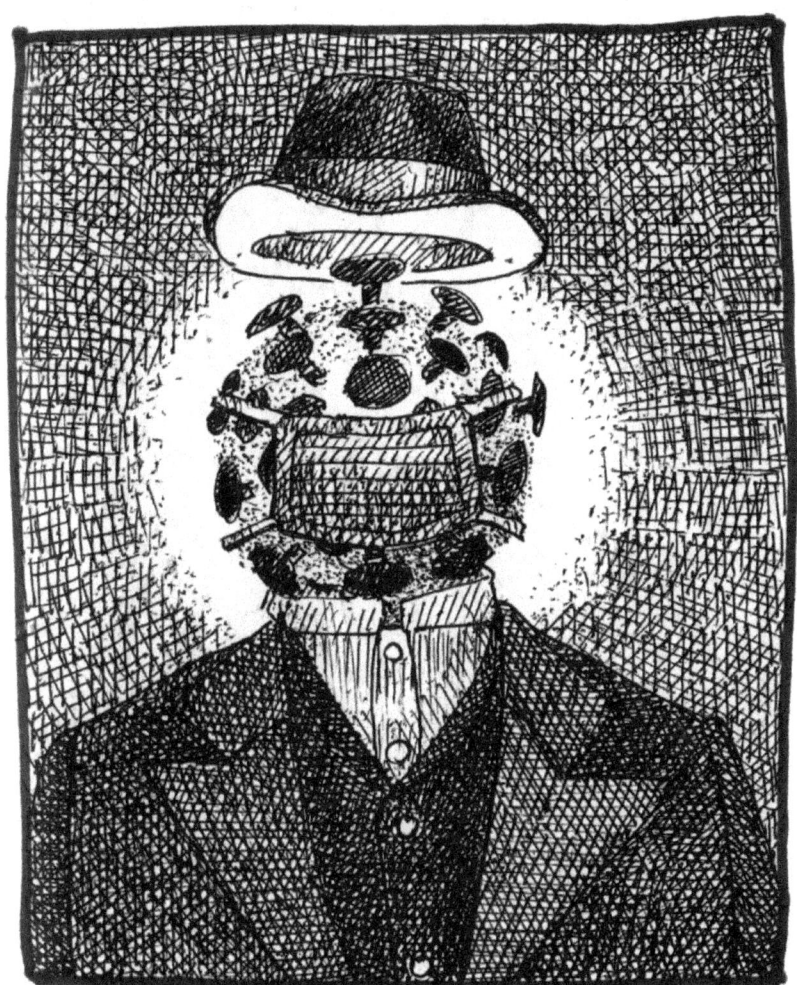

"Asymptomatic"
with Mask

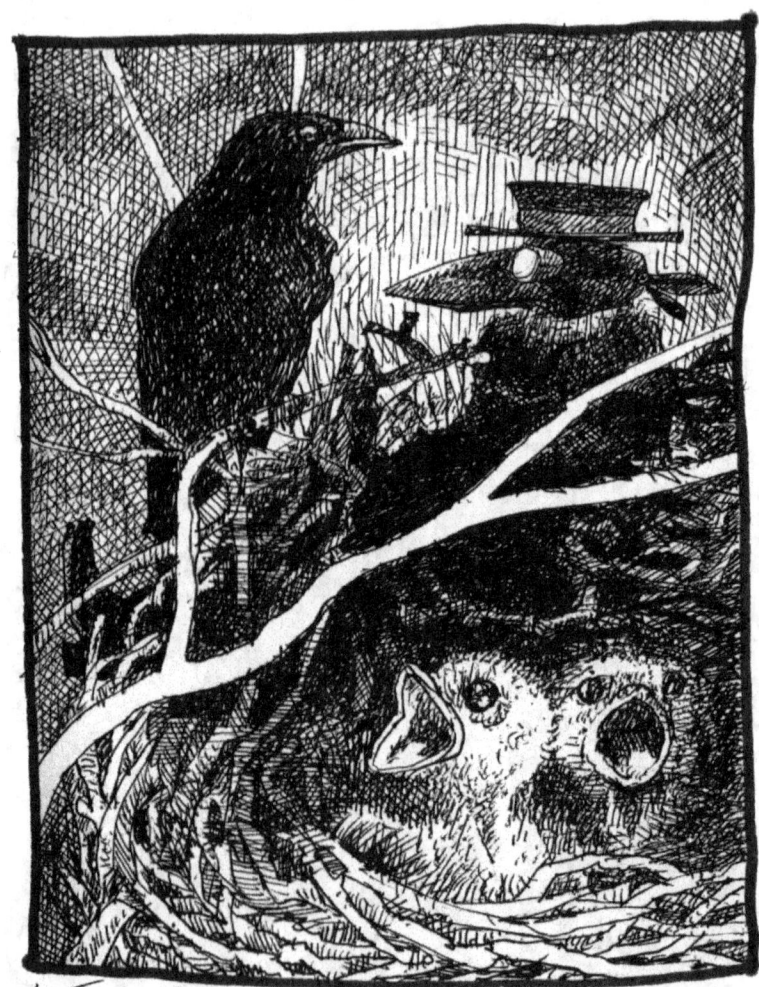

"Fledgling Plague Doctor"
Mitchell

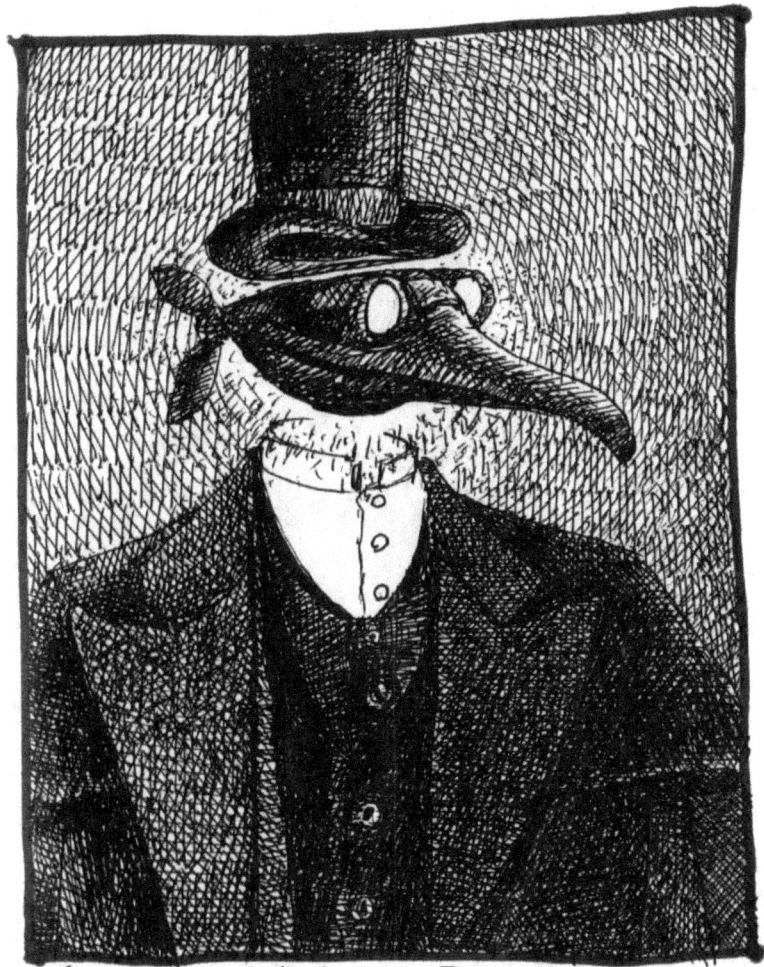

"Confident Plague Doctor"

Mitchell

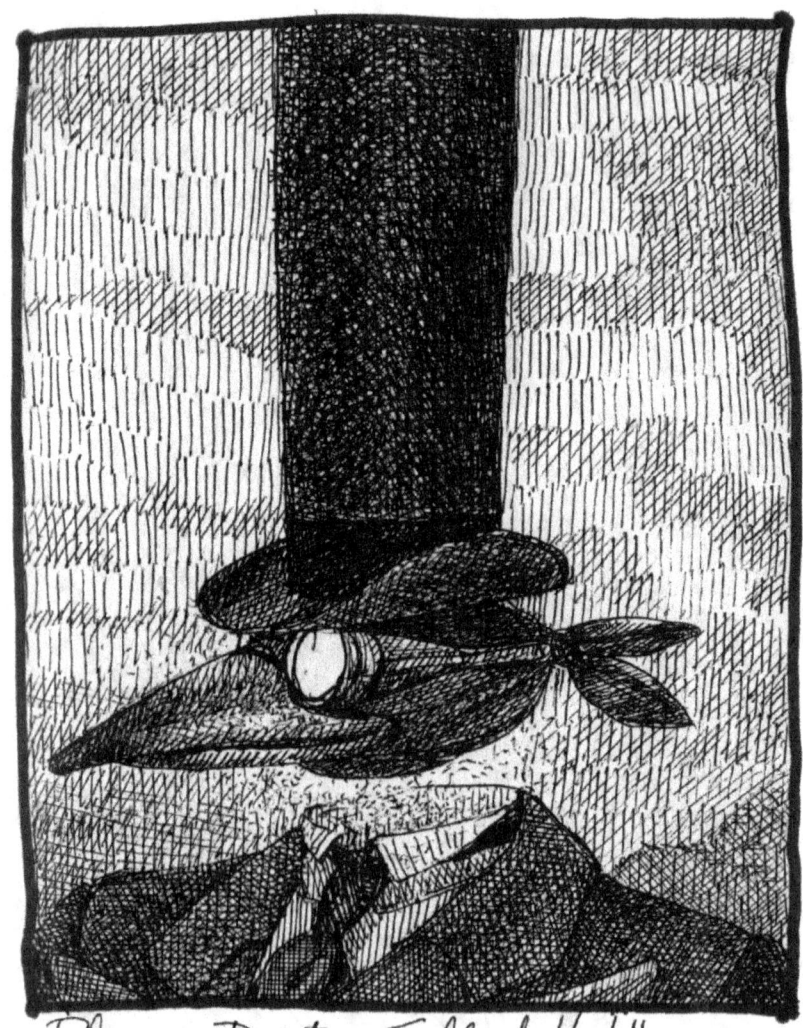

"Plague Doctor, Tallest Hat"

Mitchell

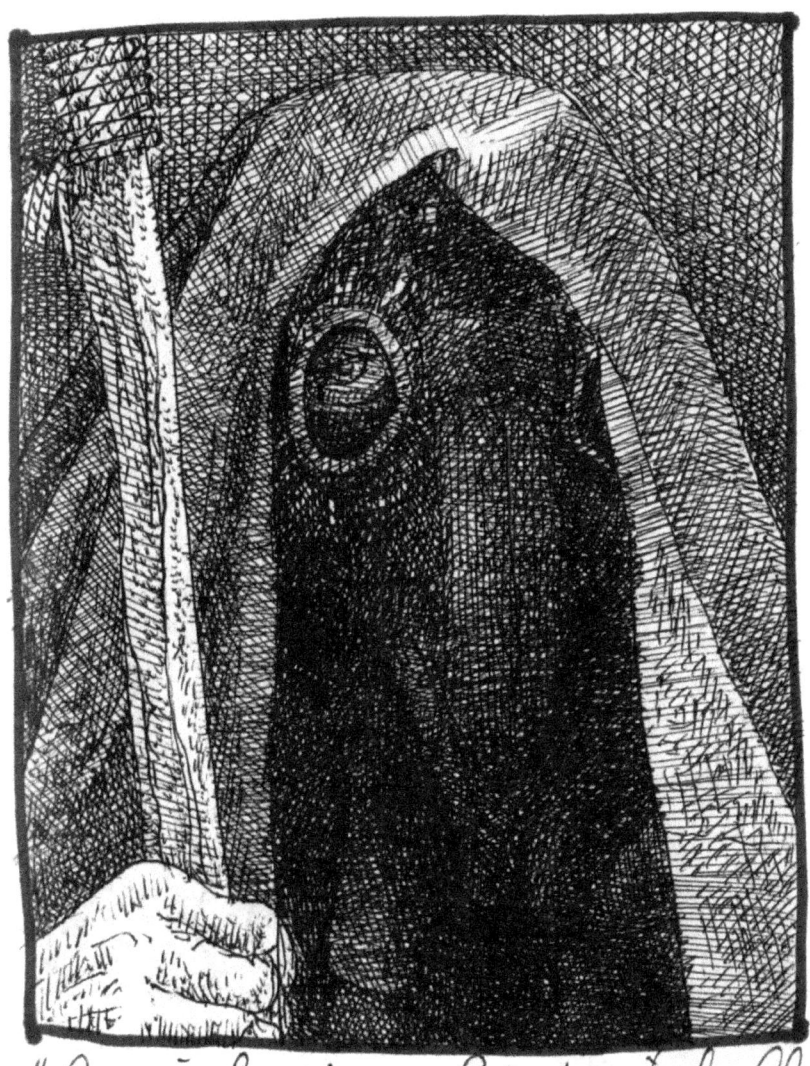

"Ancient Shroud"   Mitchell

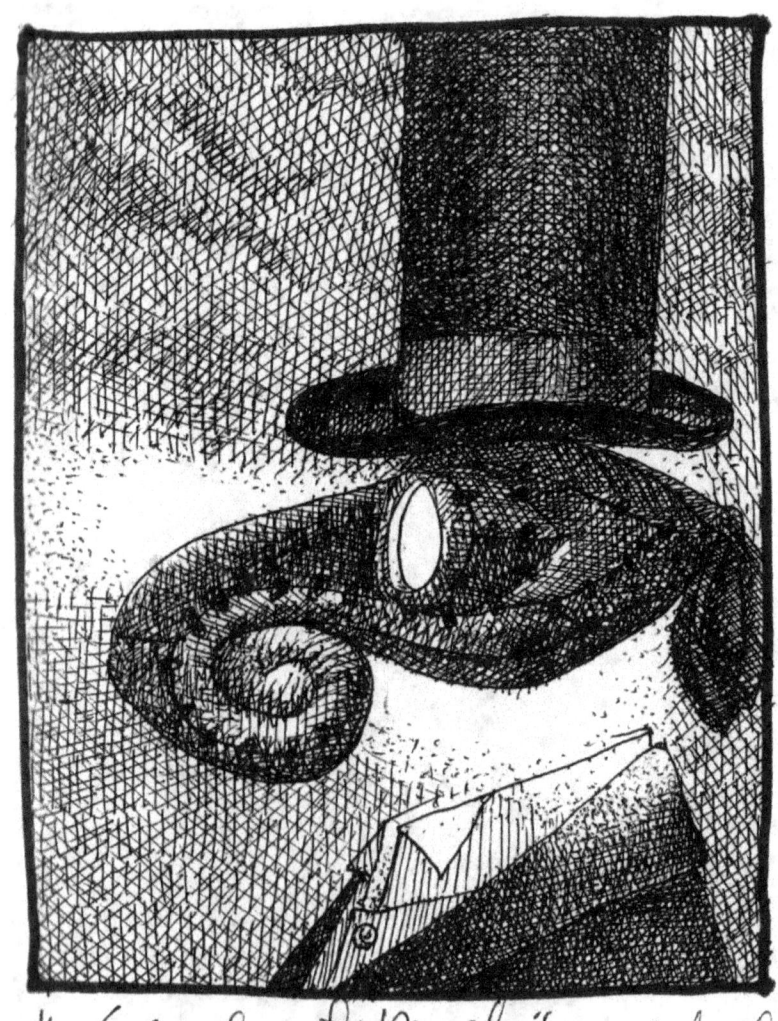

"Elephant Mask" Mitchell

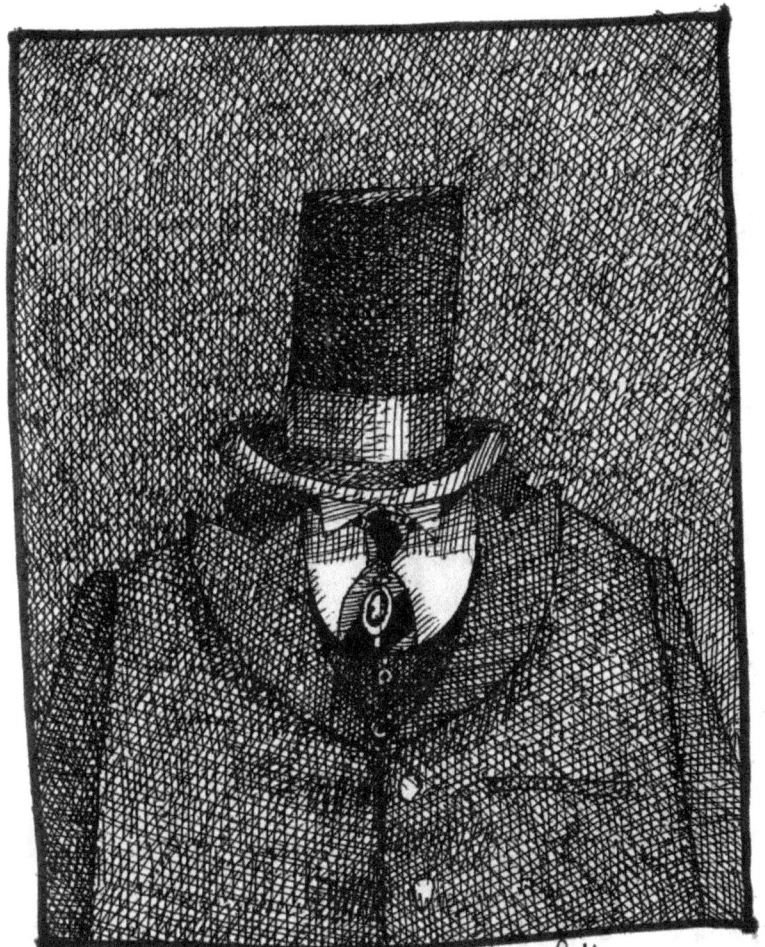

"Big Hat, Small Head" Mitchell

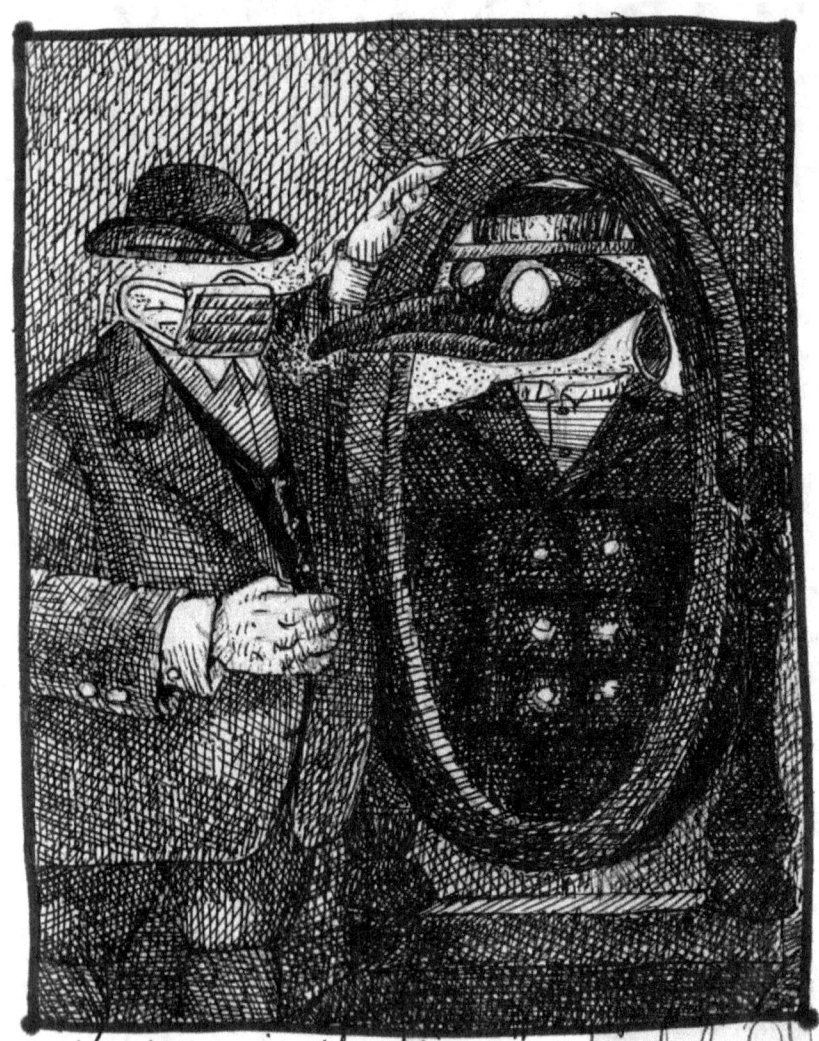

"The Man in the Mirror"   Mitchell

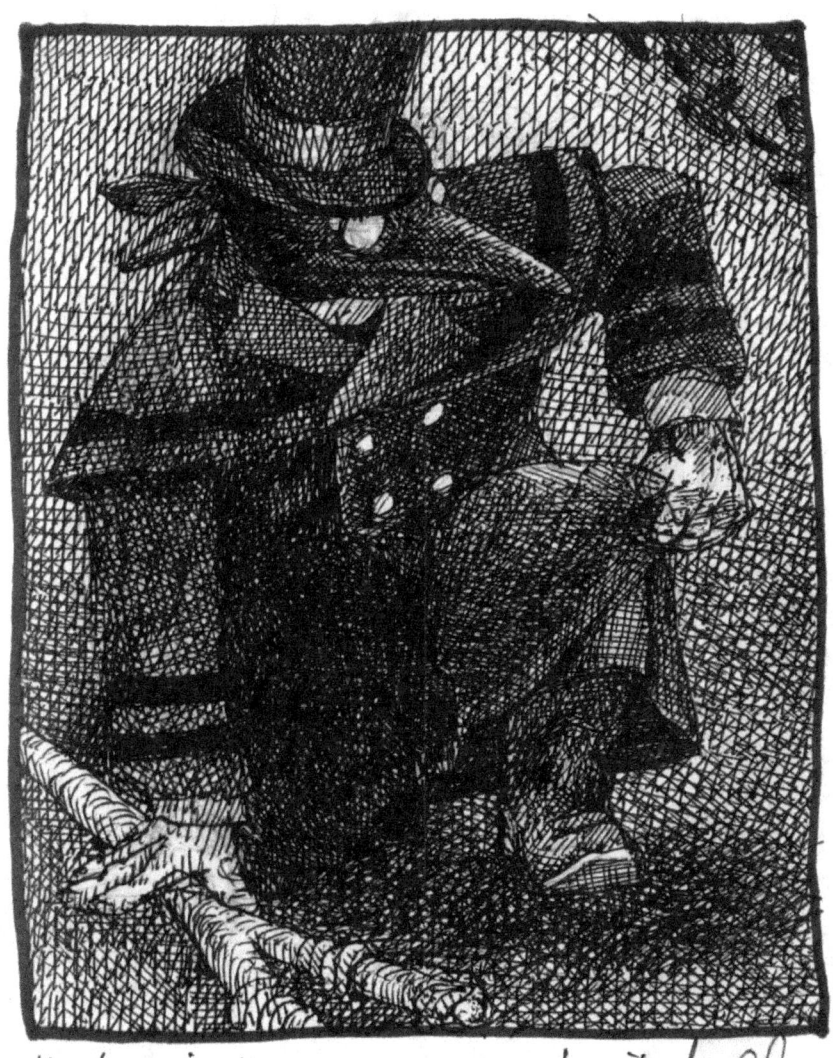

"Heroic"   Mitchell

May 29

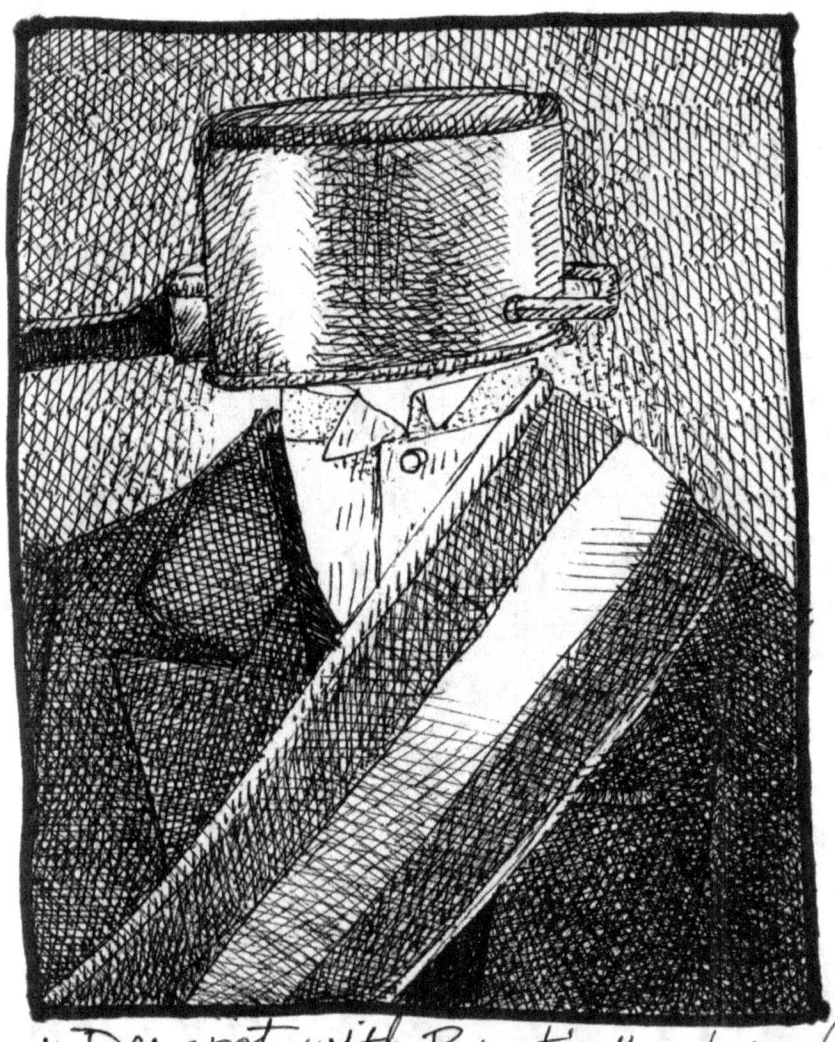

"Des-pot with Bunting" *Mitchell*

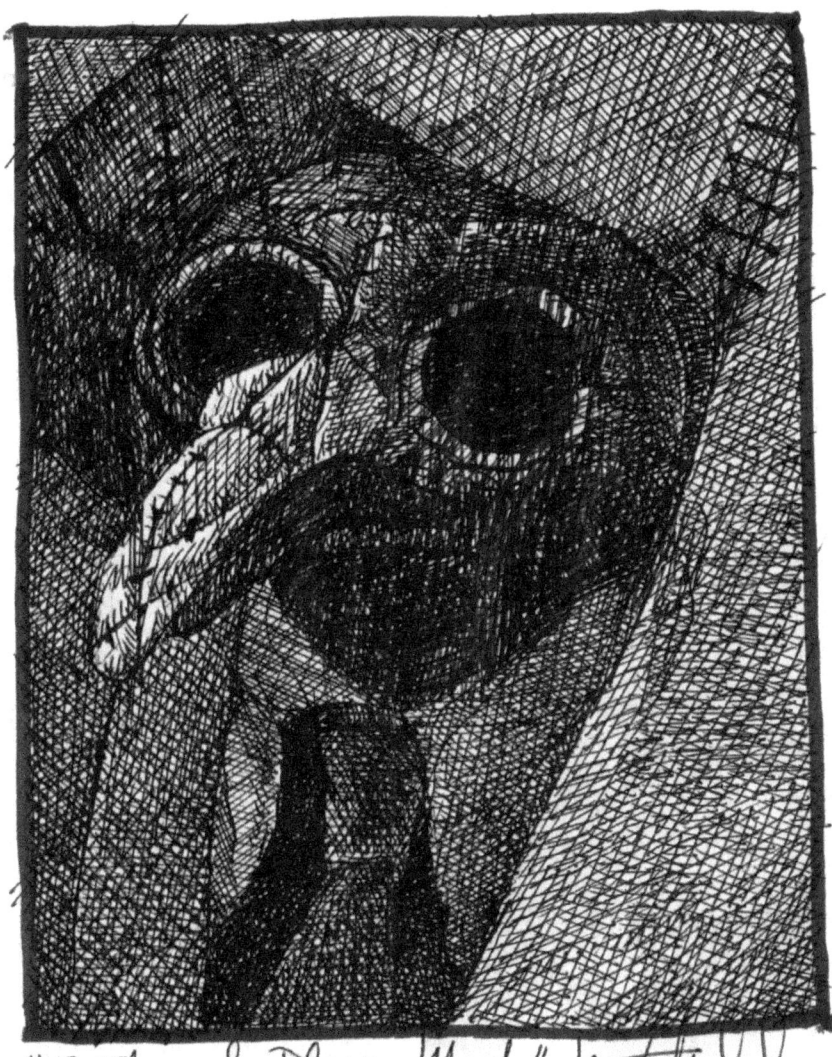

"Patchwork Plague Mask"

June 1

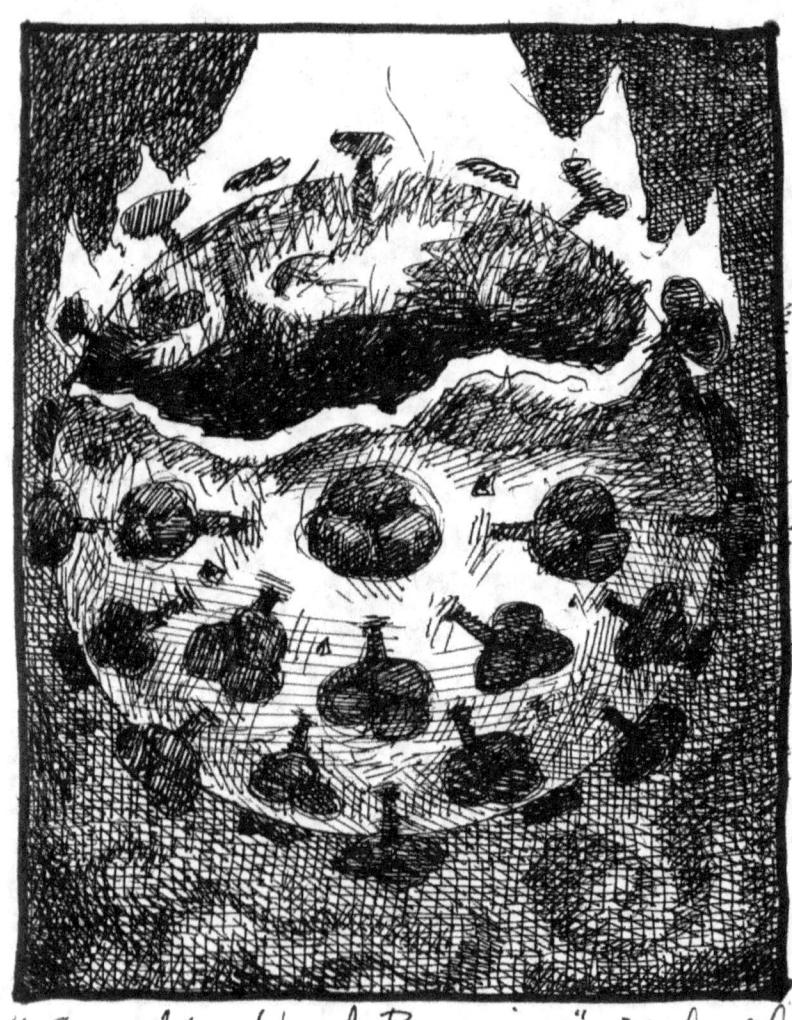

"Something Worth Burning" Mitchell

June 2

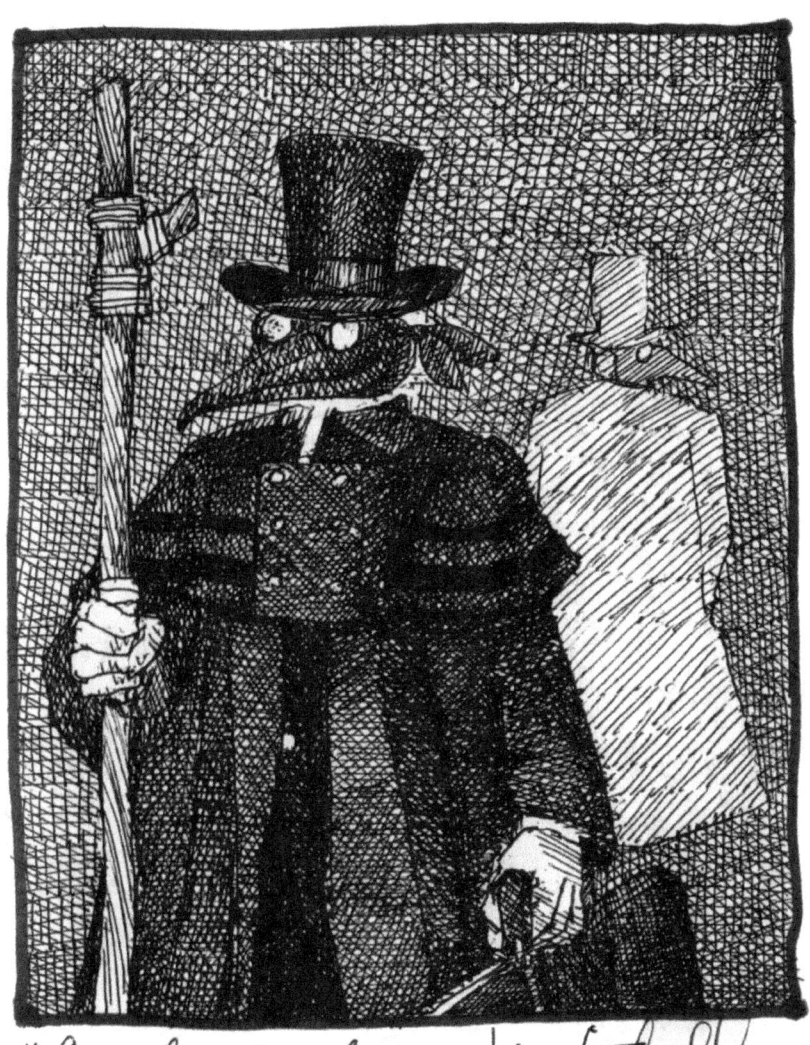

"Gotchur Back"

June 4

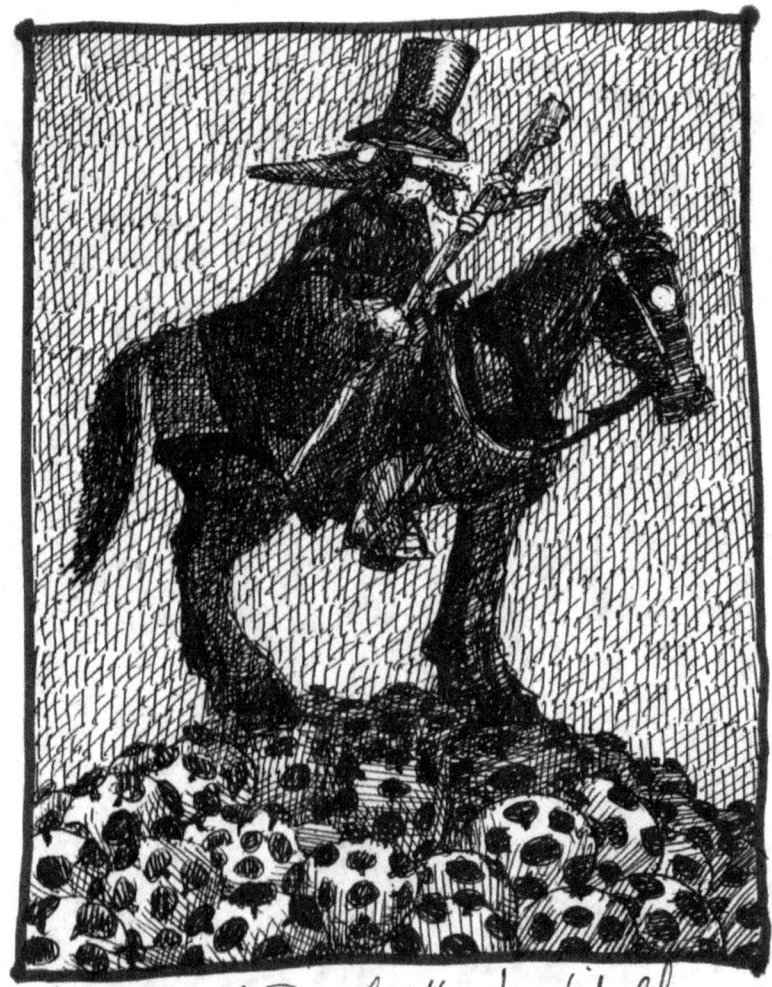

"Virus Death Dealer" Mitchell
— apologies to Frazetta

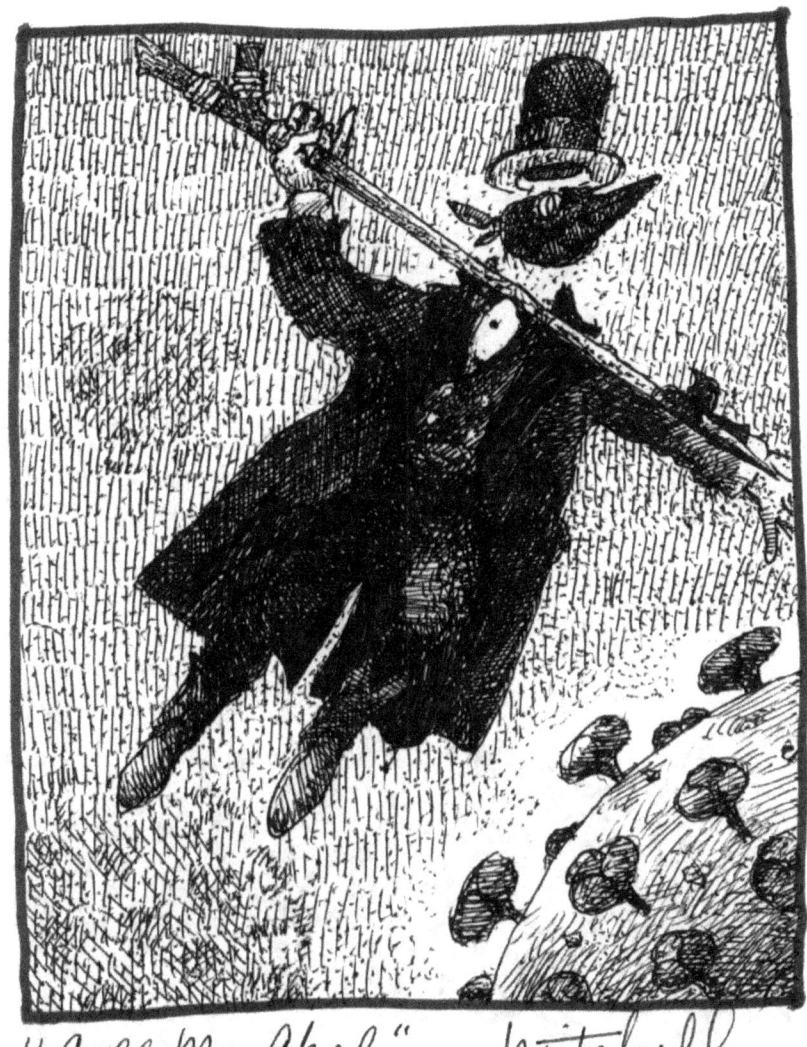

"Call Me Ahab"   Mitchell

June 11

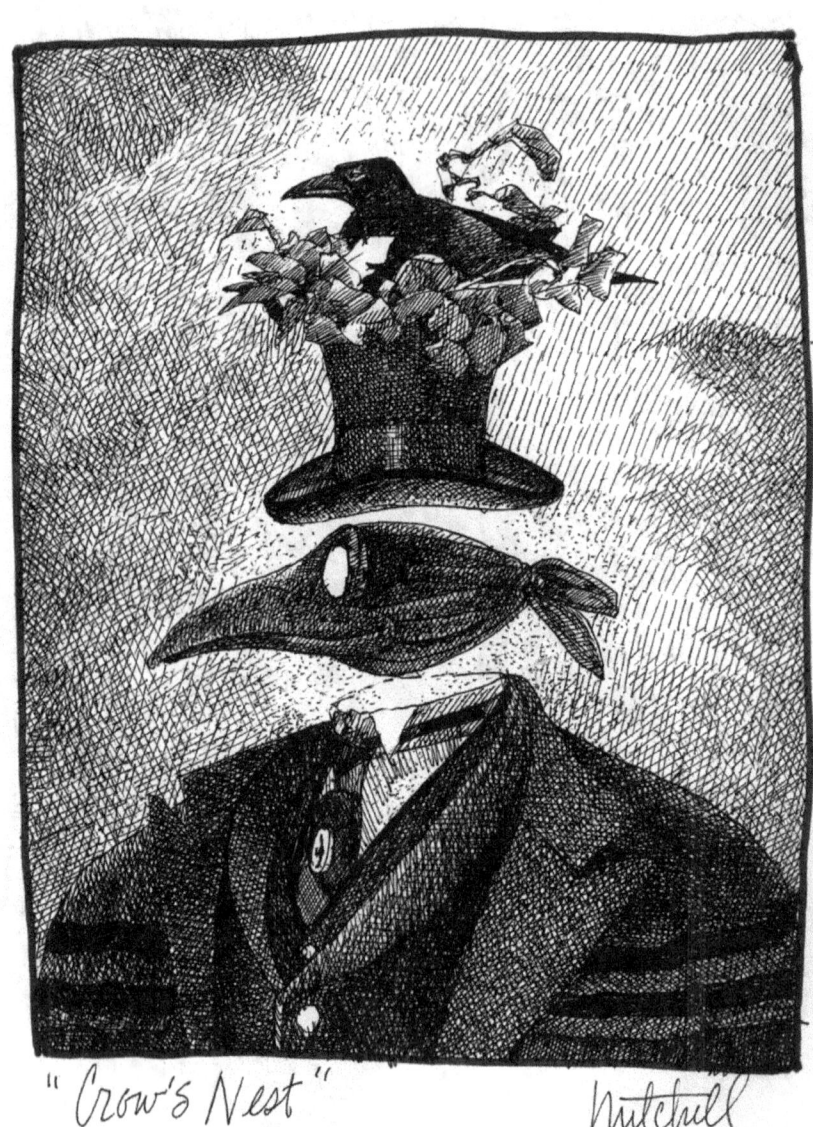

" Crow's Nest "

Mitchell

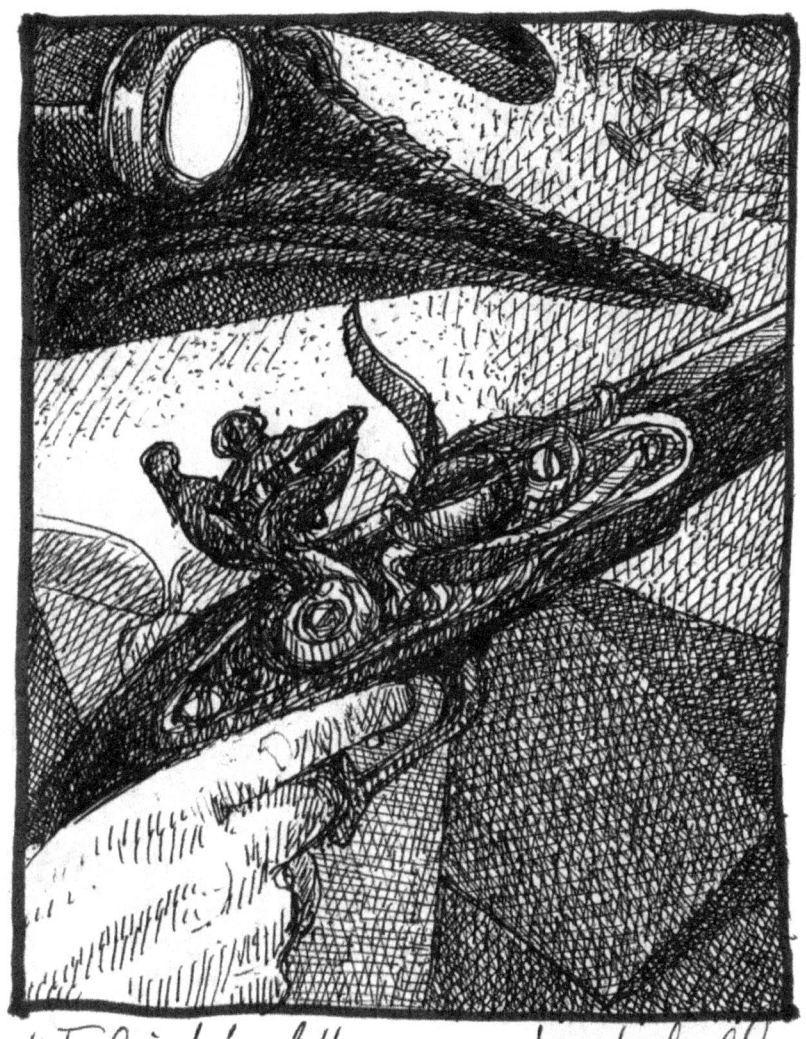

"Flintlock"   Mitchell

June 13

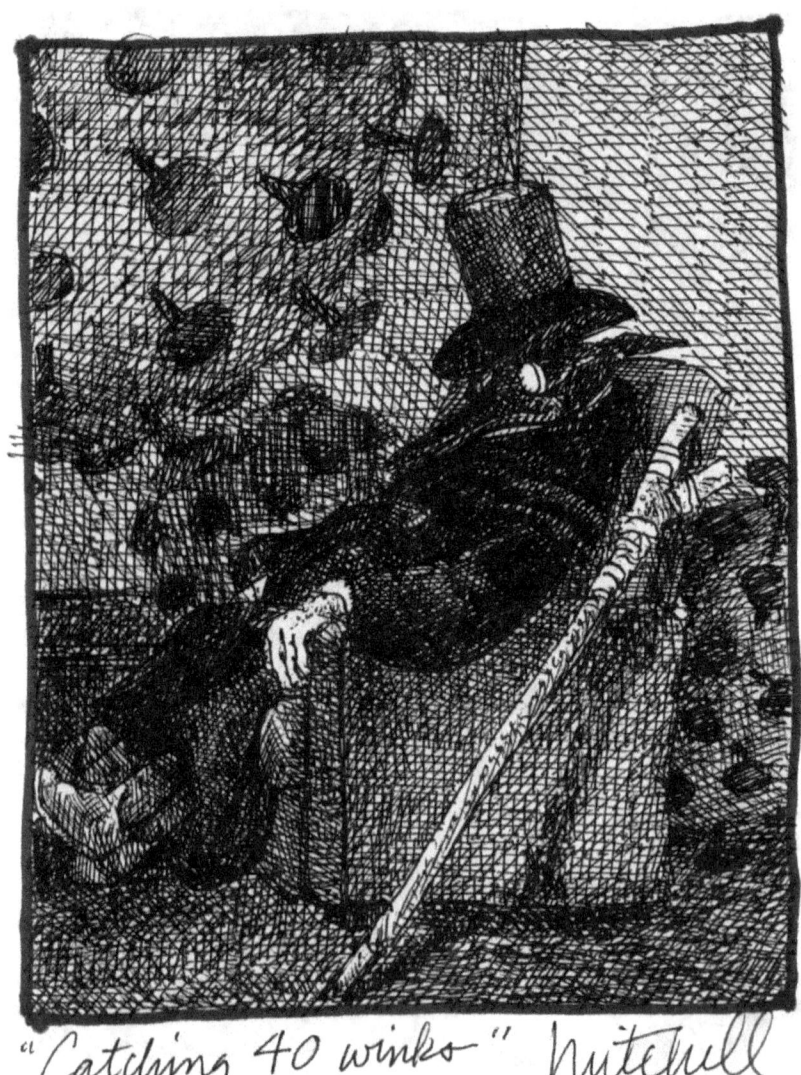

"Catching 40 winks" _Mitchell_

June 15

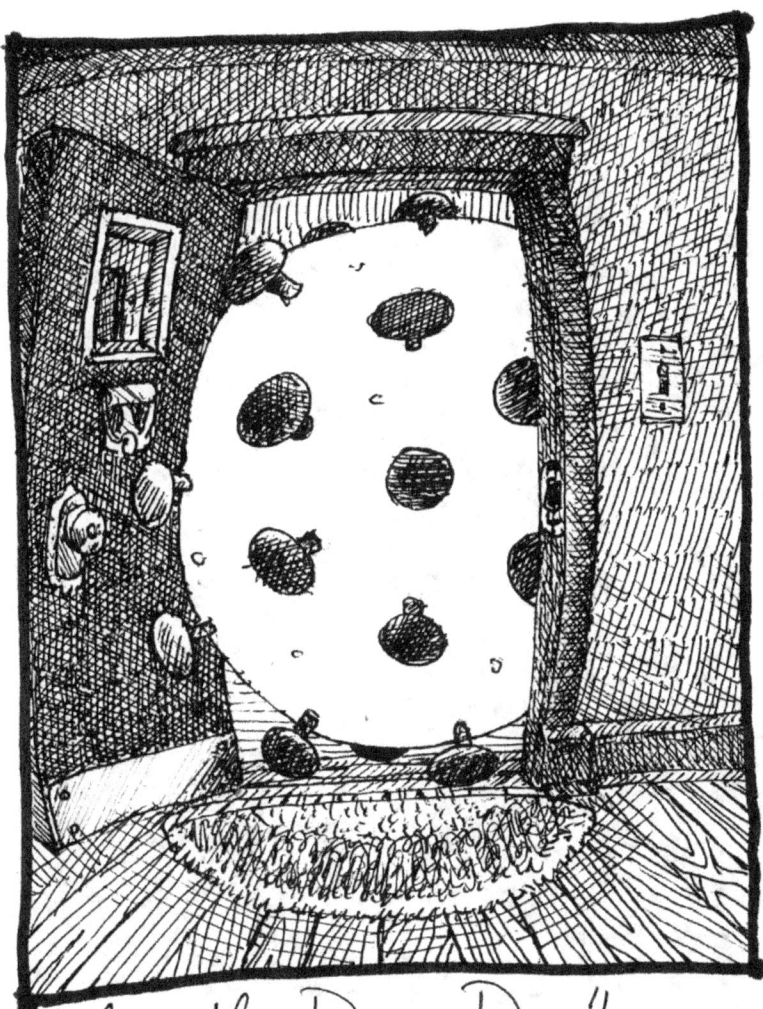

"Close the Damn Door"

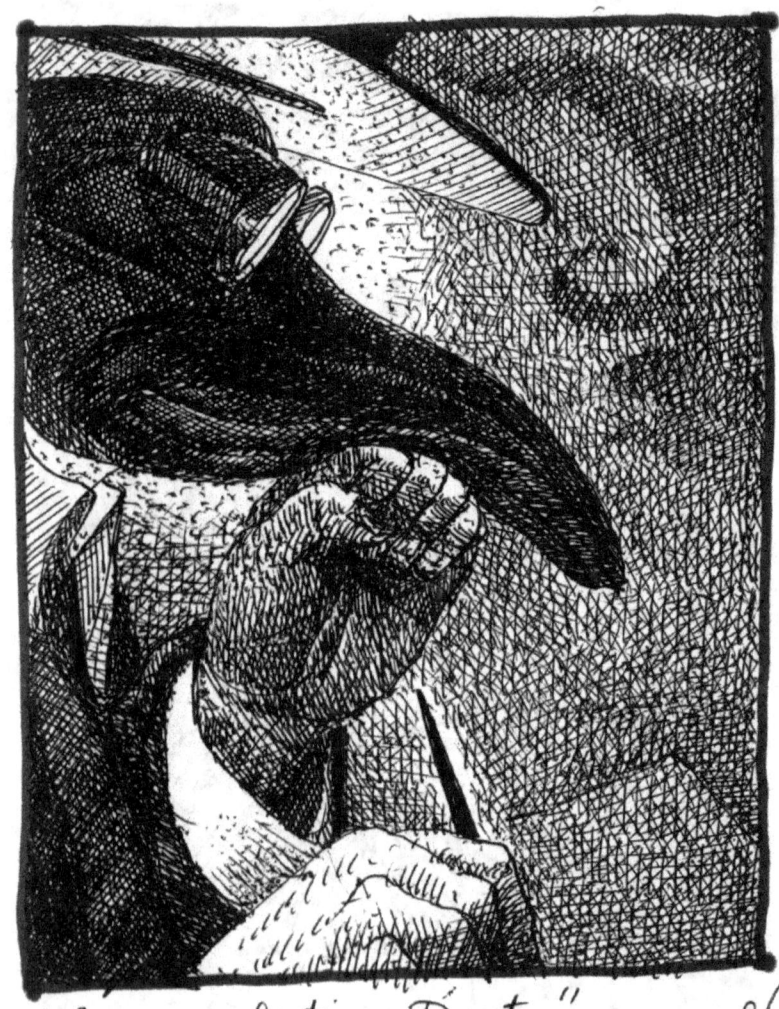

"Contemplative Doctor" Nutetulf

June 17

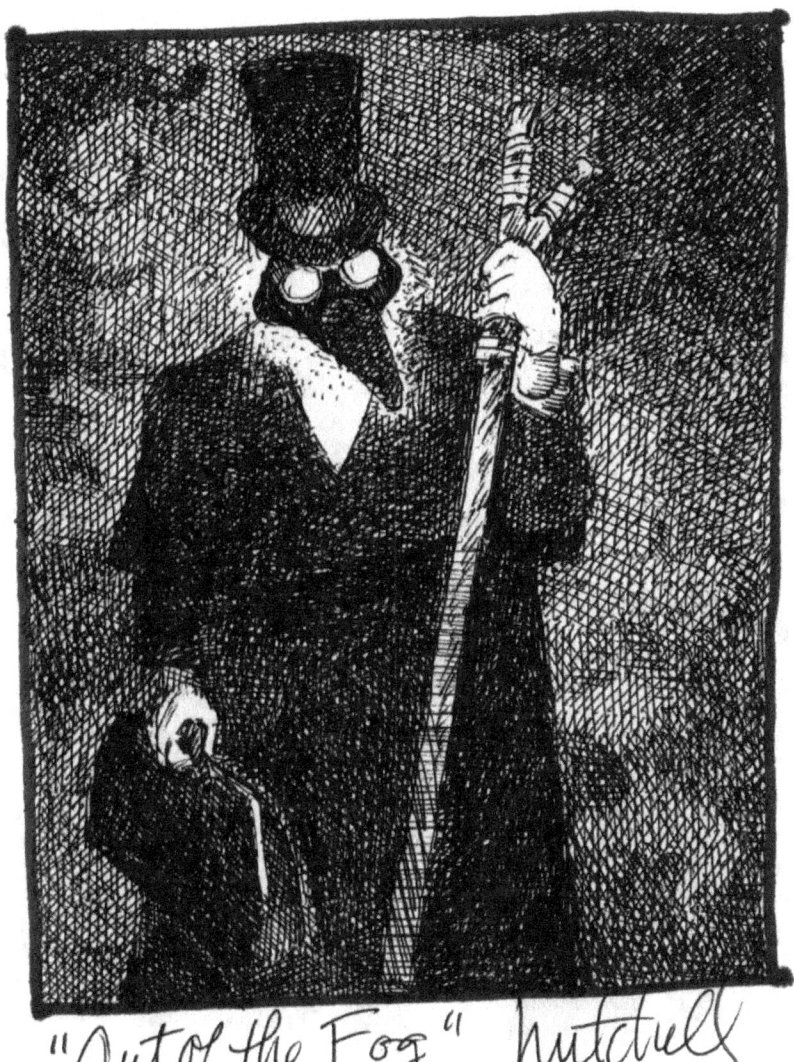

"Out of the Fog" Mitchell

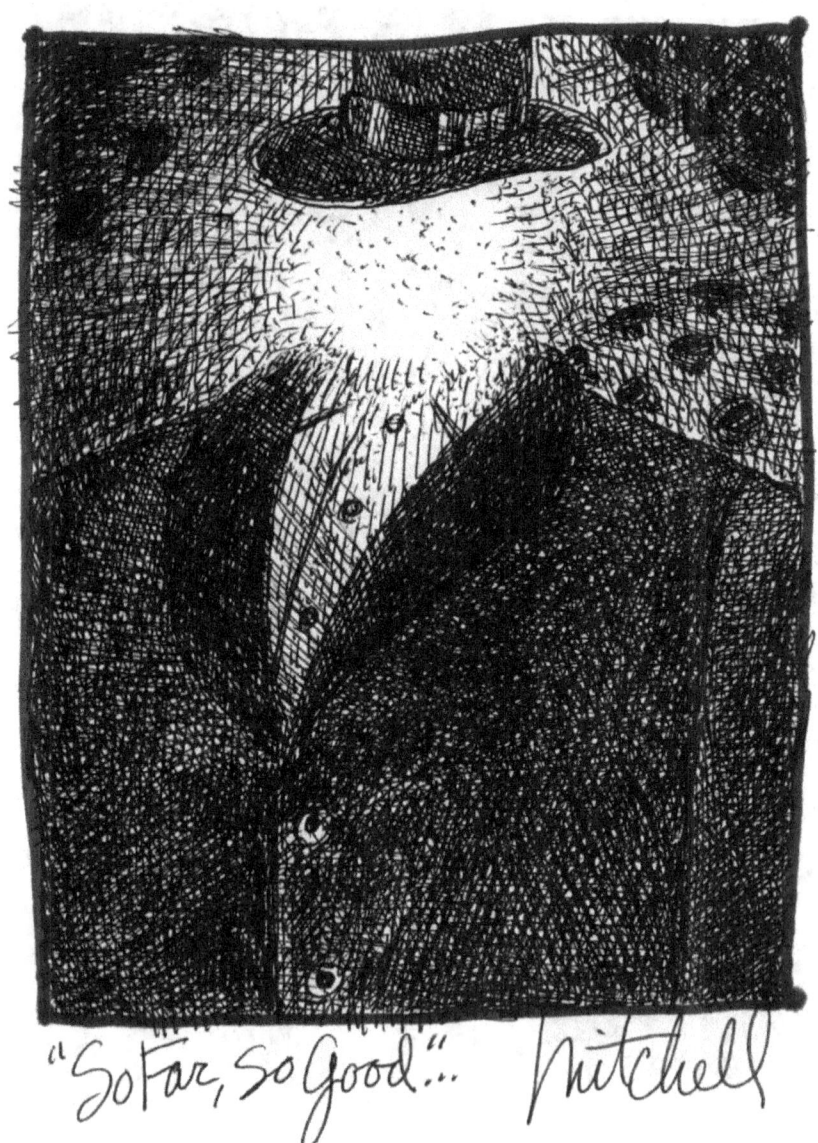

"So Far, So Good"... *Mitchell*

June 20

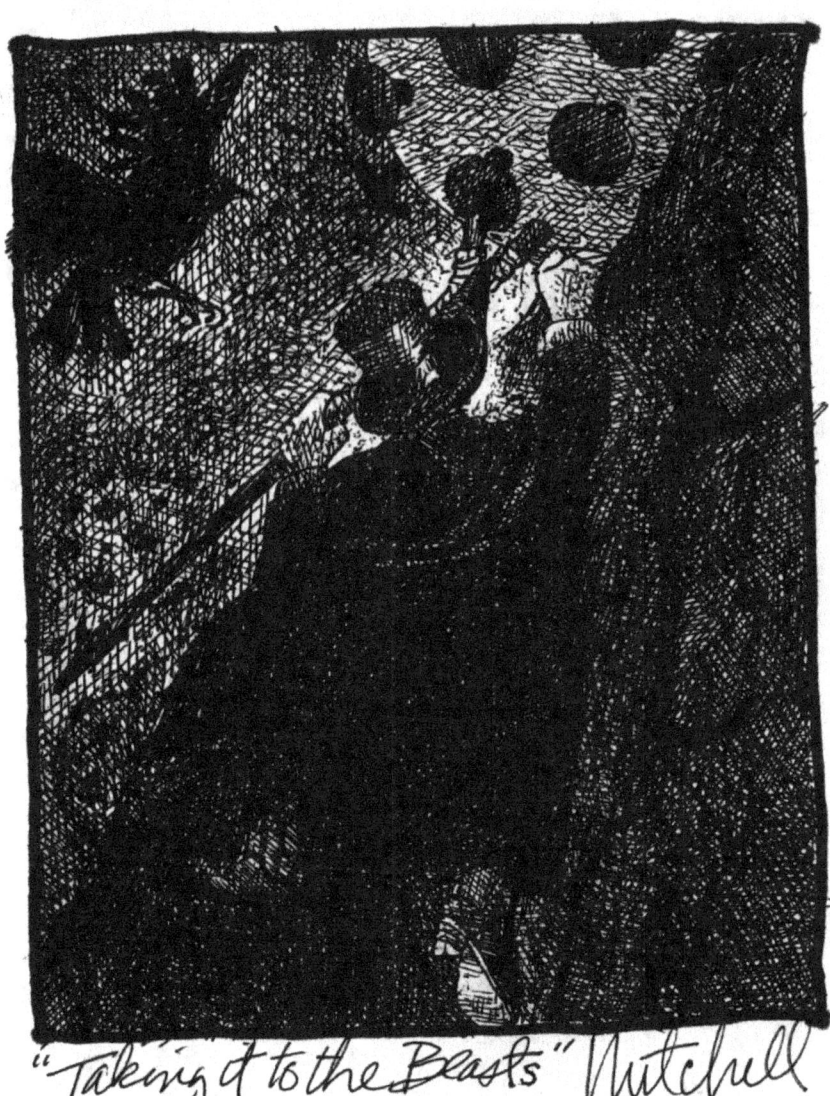

"Taking it to the Beasts" Mitchell

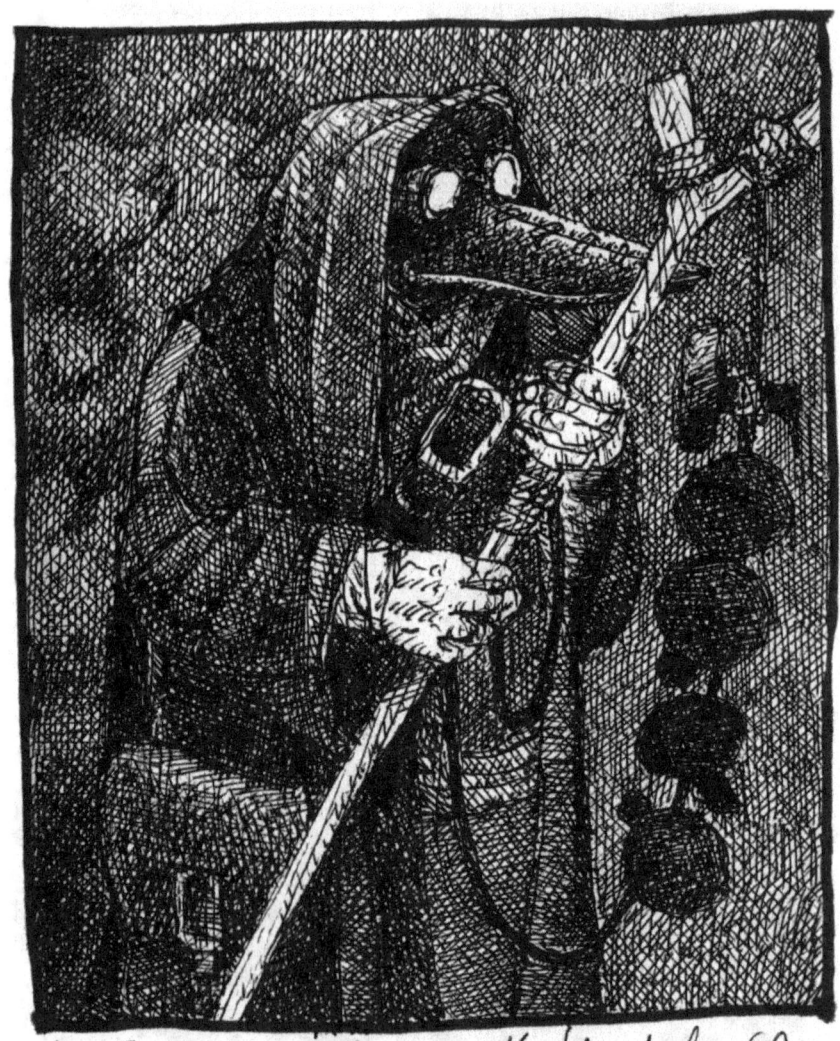

"Trophy Stringer" Mitchell

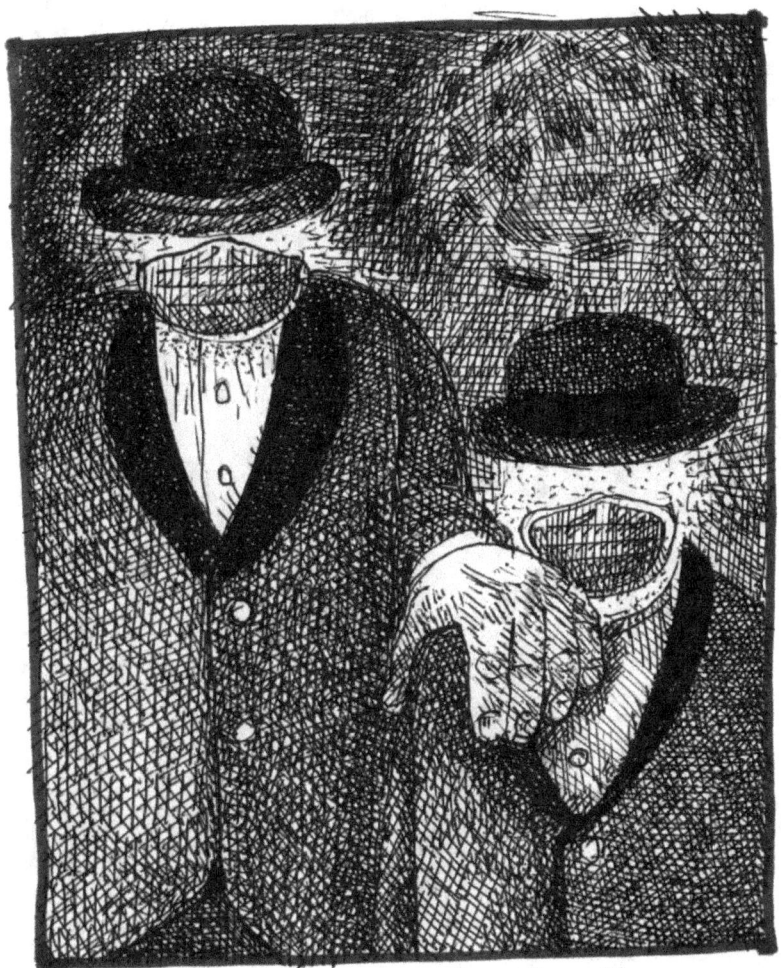

"Like Father, Like Son"

Mitchell

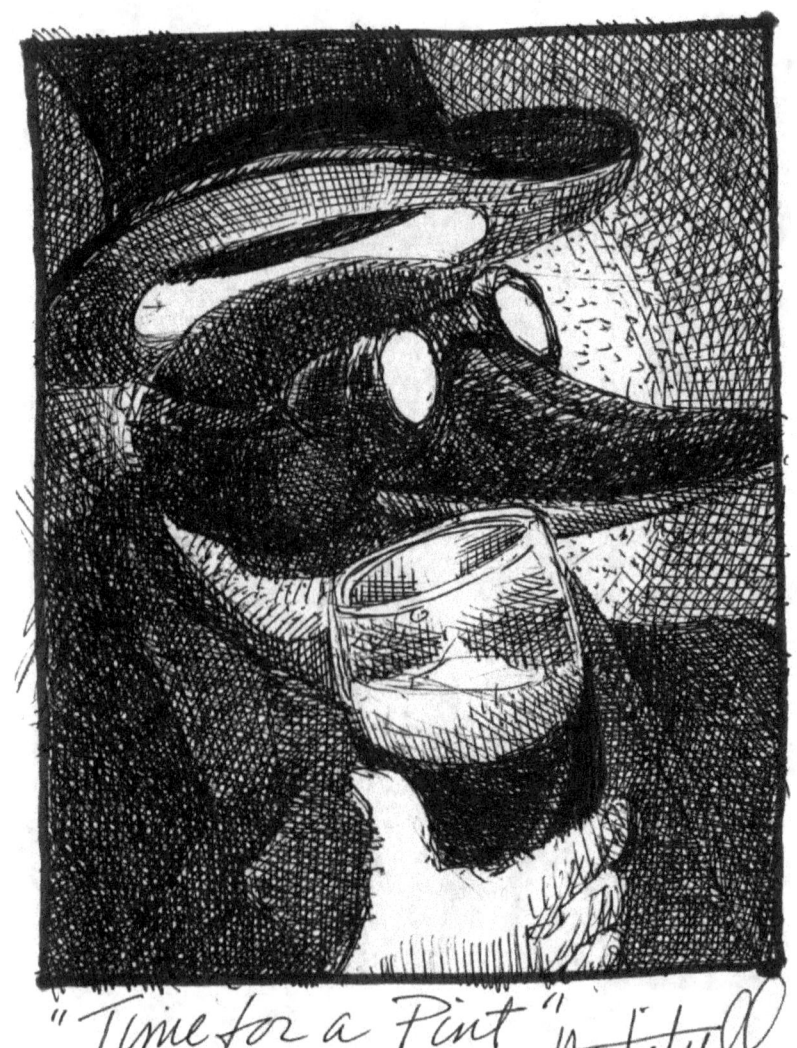

"Time for a Pint" Mitchell

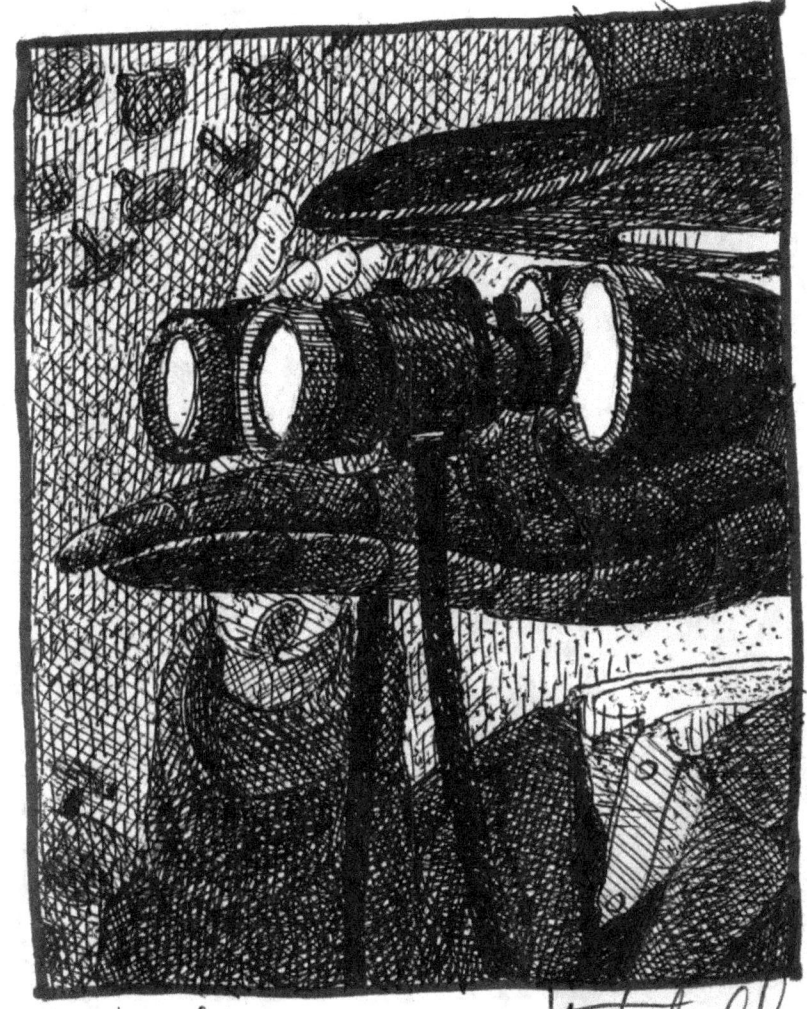

"Vigilance"

June 24

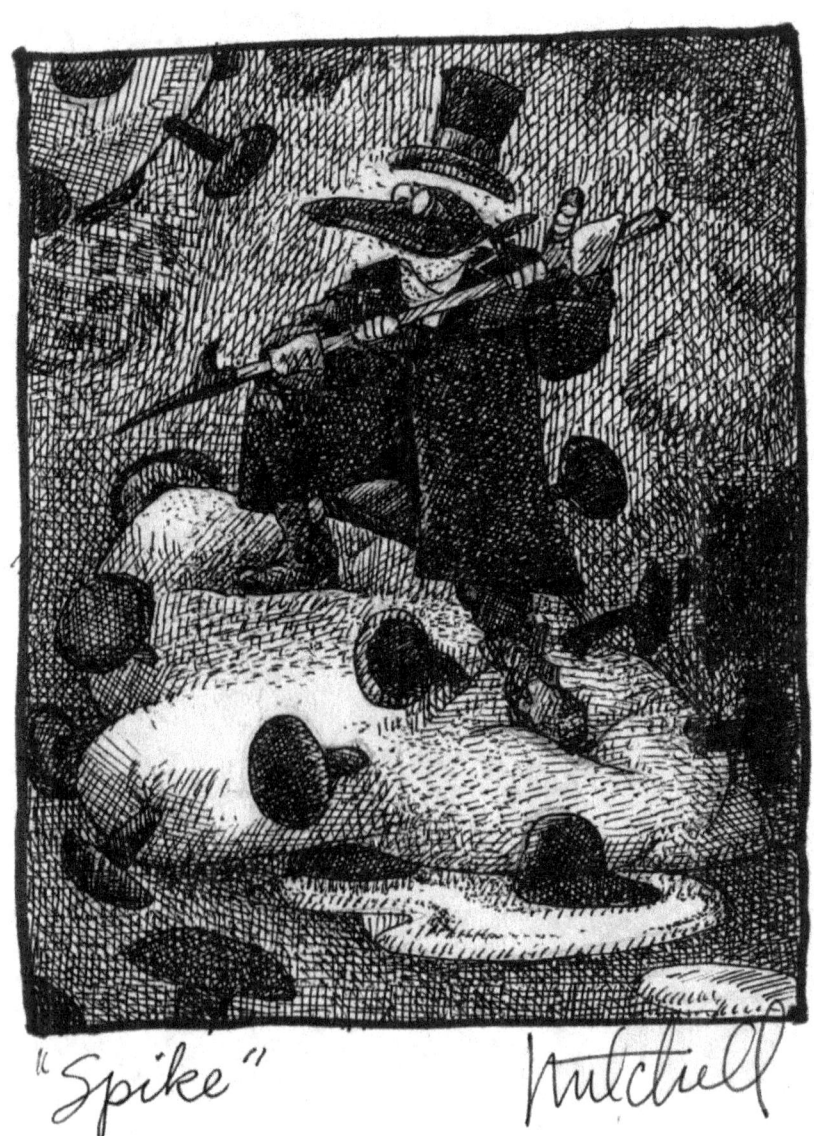

"Spike"

Mitchell

Afterword

~ Daividh Eideard Mitchell

At the end of June 2020, Kurt Mitchell died of natural causes. To say that his death was not brought on by COVID-19, however, would be incorrect. His frequent haunt, Horse Thief Hollow, which provided a major outlet for his creativity and social life, was all but shut down by the virus. The Plague Doctor series of pen & ink was his final response to the pandemic and formed a chronicle of the end of his brilliantly artistic life.

While Kurt would have undoubtedly added more plague doctors to this series, it was certain that he had plans beyond that. He had college courses to teach in the fall of 2020, whether online or in person, and more designs to contribute to Horse Thief Hollow. Clearly, Kurt didn't intend to die, and yet I take some small comfort in knowing that he was determined to make daily use of his gifts to the very end.

In the words of Horace:

> *Ask not ('tis forbidden knowledge), what our destined term of years,*
> *Mine and yours; nor scan the tables of your Babylonish seers.*
> *Better far to bear the future, my Leuconoe, like the past,*
> *Whether Jove has many winters yet to give, or this our last;*
> *This, that makes the Tyrrhene billows spend their strength against the shore.*
> *Strain your wine and prove your wisdom; life is short; should hope be more?*
> *In the moment of our talking, envious time has ebb'd away.*
> *Seize the present; trust tomorrow e'en as little as you may.*